Detecting Early Peripheral Artery Disease in Diabetic Limbs with Ultrasound Techniques

Table of Contents

Cover page..

    Title page ....

        Contents page ....

List of appendices ....

    List of tables ....

        List of figures ....

List of equations..

Acknowledgements..

    Dedication ....

        Declaration ....

Abbreviations..

book Abstract ....

Chapter 1-book Introduction 20

    1.1 What is diabetes.. 20

1.1.1 Clinical management of diabetes...22

1.1.2 Aetiology of PAD in diabetes...24

1.1.3 Classification of PAD..27

1.1.4 Beetroot juice and therapeutic management of PAD.........................29

1.2 book Rationale **33**

1.2.1 Background information...37

1.3 book aims and research questions...42

Chapter 2-Literature review 44

2.1 introduction 44

2.1.1 Methods of diagnosing PAD..45

2.1.2 Treadmill testing and six-minute walk in diagnosing PAD.......................46

2.1.3 Ankle Brachial Index in diagnosing PAD...47

2.1.4 Colour Duplex ultrasound in diagnosing PAD..48

2.2 The ultrasound parameters...51

2.2.1 Peak systolic velocity..52

2.2.2 Pulsatility Index..54

2.2.3 Vessel diameter inner to inner...55

2.2.4 Resistive Index...56

2.3 Contribution to knowledge 57

Chapter 3- book Methodology 57

3.1 book Methodology flow diagram 57

3.2 Overview of experimental research investigations 60

3.3 book experimental design..61

3.4 book inclusion and exclusion criteria...63

3.5 book recruitment strategy..66

3.6 book participants preparation...67

3.7 Body Mass Index and Ankle Brachial Index measurements...................69

3.8 Duplex ultrasound parameters measurements......................................71

3.9 Minimisation of bias and error..79

3.10 Internal and external validity...80

Chapter 4- First investigation.. 81

    Abstract..81

        4.1 Introduction 82

4.2 Aims...83

4.2.1 Research questions..83

4.3 Methodology..84

4.3.1 Design..84

4.3.2. Participants...84

4.4 Data collection procedures..85

4.4.1 Reactive hyperaemic testing...85

4.4.2 Blood tests for glycaemic control and renal function....................86

4.4.3 Doppler ultrasound parameters..87

4.4.4 Decision making during data collection...89

4.5 Statistical analysis..91

4.6 Results..93

4.6.1 Demographic findings..93

4.6.2 The Popliteal artery findings..94

4.6.3 The Anterior tibial artery findings..97

4.6.4 The posterior tibial artery findings..100

4.7 Discussion...103

4.8 Strengths and limitations..105

4.9 Conclusions and recommendations..106

4.10 Implications...107

4.11 Decision making for the second investigation....................................107

Chapter 5-Second investigation 108

   Abstract.. 108

   5.1 Introduction 109

5.2 Aims..110

5.2.1 Research questions...111

5.3 Methodology..111

5.3.1 Design..111

5.3.2 Population..112

5.3.3 Sampling..112

5.3.4 Participants..113

5.4 Data collection procedures..115

5.4.1 Recruitment plan..115

5.4.2 Duplex ultrasound parameters measurements..................................116

5.5 Statistical analysis..117

5.6 Results..118

5.6.1 Demographic findings..118

5.6.2 Confounding variable..120

5.6.3 Popliteal artery findings..121

5.6.4 Anterior Tibial Artery findings...122

5.6.5 Posterior Tibial Artery findings..124

5.7 Discussion...126

5.7.1 Duplex ultrasound parameters..126

5.7.2 Ankle Brachial Index measurements..129

5.7.3 Confounding variable...130

5.7.4 Strengths and Limitations...130

5.7.5 Internal and external validity...130

5.8 Conclusions...131

5.9 Decision making..132

5.10 Recommendations..132

Chapter 6- Third investigation 134

Abstract... 134

6.1 Introduction 135

6.2 Aim..138

6.2.1 Research questions...139

6.3 Methodology...139

6.3.1 Design..139

6.3.2 Population and sampling..140

6.3.3 Participants..140

6.4 Data collection procedures...141

6.4.1 Body Mass Index measurements..141

6.4.2 Duplex ultrasound and blood pressure measurements.................141

6.5 Statistical analysis..143

6.6 Results...145

6.6.1 Demographic Findings..145

6.6.2 Combined group changes Peak systolic velocity..........................145

6.6.3 Comparisons between groups peak systolic velocity....................147

6.6.4 Comparison within groups peak systolic velocity..........................149

6.6.5 Combined groups change systolic blood pressure......................151

6.6.6 Comparison between groups systolic blood pressure.................152

6.6.7 Comparison within groups systolic blood pressure......................153

6.6.8 Combined groups change diastolic blood pressure....................156

6.6.9 Comparison between groups diastolic blood pressure................157

6.6.10 Comparison within groups diastolic blood pressure..........................158

6.7 Discussion..160

6.8 Strengths and Limitations..164

6.9 Internal and external validity..166

6.10 Conclusions..167

6.11 Recommendations..167

6.12 Implications...167

6.13 Decision making for future research...168

Chapter 7- Overall book Discussion 169

   7.1 Introduction 169

      7.2 overall book findings 170

7.3 Overall contribution to knowledge gap..172

7.4 Overall book conclusions..173

7.5 Overall book implications..174

7.6 Overall book recommendations..175

7.8 Appendices...179

List of appendices

Appendix A: Data collection sheet investigations 1 and 2..........................179

Appendix B: Data collection sheet for both groups (Third investigation........180

Appendix C: Recruiting E-mail..181

Appendix D: Q Diabetes risk calculator...182

Appendix E1: Urea and Creatinine tests quotation......................................184

Appendix E2: Glycated haemoglobin test quotation..................................185

Appendix E3: Urea and Creatinine preliminary results................................186

Appendix E4: Glycated haemoglobin preliminary results...........................187

Appendix E5: Health professions registration Excel Laboratory....................188

Appendix F: First Investigation of raw data..189

Appendix G: UK Diabetes risk score..190

Appendix Hi): MRCZ consent form investigations 1 and 2...........................192

Appendix H ii): MRCZ Consent form third investigation..............................202

Appendix I: Sonography Principles and Instrumentation certificate.............212

Appendix J: The Abdomen and Small parts certificate...............................213

Appendix K: Obstetrics and Gynaecology certificate................................214

Appendix L: Diagnostic Radiography registration certificate......................215

Appendix M: Mpilo Hospital permission letter..216

Appendix N 1: Ultrasound practising certificate (Zimbabwe).....................217

Appendix N 2 Ultrasound registration certificate (Zimbabwe).....................218

Appendix O: MRCZ Ethics Approval letter...219

Appendix P: Rutherford et al., (1997) PAD Classification.............................220

Appendix Q1 Company Incorporation for Ultrasound centre......................221

Appendix Q2 Company incorporation for Wavestream.............................222

Appendix Q3 Health professions registration, Wavestream (PVT) LTD...........223

Appendix Q4 Tax Clearance Wavestream (PVT) LTD................................224

Appendix R MRCZ Adverse events summary..225

Appendix S1 Salford University Ethics letter...226

Appendix S2 Salford University Ethics application form...............................227

Appendix U MRCZ Acknowledgement Letter...239

Appendix W1 Brachytherapy phantom..242

Appendix W2 Brachytherapy phantom Quality control tests.....................243

List of Tables

Table 1 Health facilities profile in Zimbabwe...40

Table 2 Demographics First Investigation..94

Table 3a Descriptive statistics and DUS parameters for PA..........................95

Table 3b Descriptive statistics and paired t-tests for PA...............................96

Table 4a Descriptive statistics and DUS parameters for ATA 98

Table 4b Descriptive statistics and paired t-test for ATA...............................99

Table 5a Descriptive statistics and DUS parameters for PTA......................101

Table 5b Descriptive statistics and paired t-test for PTA.............................102

Table 6 Normality testing for demographic data..119

Table 7 confounding variable...120

Table 8 Descriptive statistics for DUS parameters both groups for PA............122

Table 9 Descriptive statistics for DUS parameters both groups for ATA...........123

Table 10 Descriptive statistics for DUS parameters both groups PTA..............125

Table 11 PSV comparisons with time...146

Table 12 SBP comparisons with time..148

Table 13 DBP comparisons with time..150

Table 14 Combined group effects SBP...151

Table 15 SBP response between groups..152

Table 16 SBP response within groups...156

Table 17 Combined groups DBP changes after BRJ....................................157

Table 18 Comparison of DBP change between groups at time points.........158

Table 19 Comparison of DBP changes at specific times within groups.........160

List of Figures

Figure 1 Administered Beetroot juice sample 33

Figure 2 Normal triphasic flow in CFA to PA..52

Figure 3 Manual trace for PSV and EDV...54

Figure 4 Blood pressure measuring technique..71

Figure 5 Measurement of Doppler parameters...75

Figure 6 scanning technique for popliteal artery 77

Figure 7 Scanning technique for anterior tibial artery..................................77

Figure 8 Lower limb arteries anatomy (CT image)..................................78

Figure 9 VDI measurements 79

Figure 10 Longitudinal section Dorsalis pedis artery..............................90

Figure 11 Longitudinal section Posterior tibial artery..............................90

Figures 12a and b PSV response to BRJ ingestion diabetics..................149

Figure 13a and b SBP response to BRJ ingestion in non-diabetics........154

Figures 14a and b DBP response to BRJ ingestion by both groups......158

List of equations

Equation 1 Pulsatility index formula..54

Equation 2 Poiseuille law..55

Equation 3 Bernoulli equation..56

Equations 4 Resistive index formula..56

Equation 5 Body Mass Index formula 69

Equation 6 Wave equation..72

Equation 7 Doppler equation..74

Equation 8 SEM Formula..93

Equation 9 SDD Formula..93

Equations 10a Sample size justification..112

Acknowledgements

A special thank you to my friends and family for their unwavering support throughout the process. Your encouragement, understanding, and patience have been the pillars that sustained me during challenging moments A special thank you to the reviewers and editors who meticulously reviewed the content, ensuring its accuracy, coherence, and overall quality.

CHAPTER 1-book introduction

This book was conducted in three experimental investigations and the first investigation aimed to firstly determine the repeatability of ultrasound parameters which include peak systolic velocity, pulsatility index, resistive index and vessel diameter inner to inner in measuring blood flow in 10 asymptomatic diabetic patients with early-stage PAD to establish their robustness before their utilisation in a larger sample size of participants in the second investigation. In the second investigation, the aim was to determine if the robust ultrasound parameters from the first investigation would able to detect the effects of early-stage PAD in the lower limb blood flow of 35 asymptomatic diabetic patients compared to 36 non-diabetic controls.
In the third investigation, the aim was to determine if the robust ultrasound parameters from the second investigation alongside systolic blood pressure (SBP) and diastolic blood (DBP) would be able to show the acute effects of ingested beetroot juice by the same sample of participants from the second investigation.

In this chapter, the first outline is an overview of the main pathological process being researched in this book which is Type 2 diabetes and its complication of peripheral arterial disease (PAD) in the lower limb arteries, followed by the overview of the current methods of imaging PAD and therapy then finally the rationale which prompted the undertaking of this book.

1.1   What is Diabetes Mellitus?

Diabetes is a highly oxidative and inflammatory process which encompasses a group of pathologies which cause various disorders of metabolism, which is mainly caused by either non-secretion of the hormone insulin by the pancreas (Type I diabetes) or insulin resistance which refers to the body's inability to effectively use the secreted hormone insulin (Type II diabetes) to enable sufficient metabolism of glucose, which in turn results in hyperglycaemia and the increased metabolism of fats and proteins (Steinberg, 2009; Steinberg and Wizturn 2010; Jude 2014; Kaku 2010).

Type 1 Diabetes Mellitus manifests following the destruction of pancreatic β-cells either due to idiopathic causes or autoimmune reactions in the pancreas. This results in a total deficiency of insulin for glucose metabolism, however, Type 2 Diabetes Mellitus is a heterogeneous disorder caused by a combination of genetic factors related to the impaired insulin secretion, insulin resistance and environmental factors such as obesity, overeating, lack of exercise, stress and ageing (Kaku, 2010; Bhatia et al., 2004) in particular people aged over 30 years but evidence has indicated it increasing in younger people (less than 30 years) especially the obese (Seino et al., 2010; Biswas et al., 2006). Evidence has also indicated a positive correlation between parental history of diabetes and the gradual manifestation of its symptoms such as reduced insulin secretion in the offspring of such parents (Vaukhonen et al., 2000) and lifestyle factors like overweight, and higher levels of triglycerides (Chen et al., 2012; Sun et al., 2013; Type 2 Diabetes in adults: management (NG 28) NICE, 2018; Macleod et al., 2008).

Confirmation of chronic hyperglycaemia is essential for the diagnosis of Type 2 Diabetes Mellitus and it is concluded if there is a fasting plasma glucose level of greater or equal to 126 mg/dl (greater or equal to 70 mmol/l), a glycated haemoglobin level of greater or equal to 7 %, Albumin: Creatinine ratio of greater or equal to 30 mg/g and microalbuminuria greater or equal to 20 µg/min (Seino et al., 2010; Sun et al., 2013; Biswas et al., 2006). Type 2 Diabetes is commonly associated with raised blood pressure, disturbed blood lipid levels and a tendency to develop thrombosis thus an increased risk for cardiovascular diseases (Kiboki et al., 2000; Zeng et al., 2000; Kim et al., 2001). Prior evidence (Norgren et al., 2007; Yoshimura et al., 2006) has also indicated that each 1% increase in glycated haemoglobin results in a 25 % increase in the risk of PAD.

1.1.1 Clinical Management of Type 2 Diabetes Mellitus.

Some countries, such as the United Kingdom (UK) and United States of America (USA), have well developed national guidelines on the management and treatment of Type 2 Diabetes in adults (16 - 68 years), and the guidelines are current, evidence-based and patient-centred (Type 2 Diabetes in adults: management (NG28), NICE, 2015; Eisenstein et al., 2017; Rooke et al., 2011). However, according to the National Strategy of Zimbabwe's health delivery system for 2016-2020, it was noted that currently Zimbabwe has not yet implemented policies which strengthen the utilisation of global guidelines on the management of Type 2 Diabetes and other communicable diseases across the country and there was advocacy for these guidelines to be implemented (Parirenyatwa and Gwinji, 2016; Hakim et al., 2005). The UK and USA guidelines of Type 2 Diabetes management in adults were designed to be easily understood by the healthcare professionals, the diabetic patients as well as their families and carers while they are availed at primary care level (Carthy 2013; Eisenstein et al., 2017; Hirsch et al., 2005; Rooke et al., 2011). These guidelines have been tailored in a systematic approach which supports patients' change of behaviour in the following aspects;

i) Healthy life choices which include healthy eating, physical activity, tobacco cessation, weight management and effective ways to cope with stress.

ii) Self-management of disease which includes self-monitoring for blood pressure which should be maintained at least below 140/80 mmHg and below 130/80 mmHg if there is kidney, eyes or cerebral disease.

iii) Glucose monitoring which should be maintained as glycated haemoglobin levels (HbA$_{1c}$) 53 mmol/l (7.0%), while antiplatelet therapy is offered as Aspirin or Clopidogrel) but will not be prescribed for patients without cardiovascular disease.

iv) Prevention of diabetes complications which include self-monitoring for foot health, active participation in screening for eyes, feet, kidneys and immunisations.

v) Identification of self-management problems and develop strategies to solve these problems including self-selected behavioural goal setting.

vi) Treatment options include firstly a standard release Metformin as the initial drug treatment, and where metformin is contraindicated or not tolerated, initial drug treatment with dipeptidyl peptidase-4 of a Sulfonylurea will be considered.

Clinical management for patients with type 2 diabetes at Mpilo hospital diabetic clinic in Zimbabwe utilises Sliding Scale insulin (SSI) method and according to the Colunga-Lozano et al., (2018), the SSI method refers to increasing administration of premeal insulin dose based on the blood sugar level before the meal. The following steps are undertaken in the management of diabetic patients at Mpilo hospital in Zimbabwe;

i) Random blood sugar testing is done on the patients as they present to the clinic,

ii) If the random sugar levels signal hyperglycaemia which reflects as greater than 20 mmol/l the patient would be admitted in the hospital.

iii) The patient is put on an insulin injection which is offered on a sliding scale thus matching the level of hyperglycaemia in the patient (Colunga-Lozano et al., 2018).

iv) Glycated haemoglobin levels (HbA_{1c}) tests are ordered though limited by affordability by most patients, and if again these tests are found to be indicating hyperglycaemia which reflects as HbA_{1c} greater or equal to 7% then insulin is offered on a sliding scale as follows;

Above 16% HbA$_{1c}$	12 units Insulin
12 – 16% HbA$_{1c}$	8 units Insulin
8 – 12% HbA$_{1c}$	4 units Insulin
HbA$_{1c}$ <8%	nothing is prescribed.

v) During the first 24 – 48 hrs, Urea and electrolyte tests would be ordered to assess the preserved renal function.

vi) If Estimated Glomerular Filtration Rate is above 45 ml/min/1, 74 m the patient is prescribed on oral medication mostly Metformin drugs as backbone therapy.

vii) The patient is admitted at least for 10 days in the hospital and they then receive counselling about healthy eating, feet care and the wearing of comfortable shoes, exercising and stopping smoking.

viii) No antiplatelet therapy is offered yet in these patients.

1.1.2 Aetiology of peripheral artery disease (PAD) in Diabetic patients.

In the endothelial cells of arterial walls under normal circumstances insulin stimulates the expression and activity of endothelial nitric oxide synthase, resulting in increased production of nitric oxide which is critical for the process of vasodilation, thus maintaining stable blood pressure in the human body (Kiboki et al., 2000; Zeng et al., 2000; Kim et al., 2001). Endothelial nitric oxide is also part of the antioxidant defence system responsible for clearing reactive oxygen species, low-density lipoproteins and free radicals which are mostly produced during a host of defence and immunologic reactions by activated macrophages, thus retarding the rate of atherogenesis (Steinberg, 2009; Steinberg and Wizturn, 2010).

Insulin also promotes and maintains vascular smooth muscle cells in a well-differentiated and contractile state, thus reducing the chances of proliferation due to poor differentiation by these cells in its absence (Kiboki et al., 2000; Zeng et al., 2000; Kim et al., 2001). These stimulatory effects of insulin on Endothelial

Nitric Oxide Synthase and nitric oxide production are therefore equally important in preventing endothelial dysfunction and early pro-atherosclerotic changes which lead to PAD (Kiboki et al., 2000; Zeng et al., 2000; Kim et al., 2001).

Peripheral Artery Disease is thus defined as atherosclerosis of the distal aorta and lower limb arteries causing arterial narrowing and impairment of blood circulation to the legs and diabetes is one of the main risk factors for causing PAD besides smoking hypertension and dyslipidaemia (Sun et al., 2013; Type 2 Diabetes in adults: management (NG 28), NICE, 2015).

The chronic absence of insulin in diabetic patients also leads to a chronic absence of nitric oxide resulting in high blood pressure, dyslipidaemia, high levels of Reactive Oxygen Species, Low-Density Lipoproteins and free radicals in the circulation resulting in a gradual build-up of plaque and narrowing of arterial walls (Steinberg, 2009; Steinberg and Wizturn, 2010; Boaz et al., 2000), thus diabetes accelerates and worsens the occurrence of atherosclerosis increasing the risks of cardiovascular complications such as stroke, retinopathy, nephropathy and peripheral artery disease to mention a few. Such complications constitute the main causes of poor prognosis amongst diabetic patients if left untreated (Seino et al., 2010).

Peripheral arterial disease is therefore defined as atherosclerosis of the distal aorta and lower limb arteries causing arterial narrowing and impairment of blood circulation to the legs. Diabetes follows smoking as one of the main risk factors for PAD, besides hypertension and dyslipidaemia (Sun et al., 2013; Jude, 2004; Peihua, 2003). This process of atherogenesis progresses gradually in diabetic patients, even though most of them may be asymptomatic within the early stages (Sun et al., 2013; Peihua, 2003). However, lack of symptoms may not always be linked with early-stage PAD for evidence has shown lack of symptoms in diabetic patients with late-stage PAD especially if they experience neuropathy or lead lives of inactivity (Sun et al., 2013; Jude, 2004).

According to a study by Fowkes et al., (2013), PAD was shown as the third leading cause of atherosclerotic cardiovascular morbidity after coronary artery disease and stroke both in high income and low to medium-income countries. Gender-specific prevalence rates of PAD were found to increase with age and the prevalence in high-income countries in men at 45 – 49 years was 5.28% (95% CI, 3.38 - 8.17) while in women it was 18.83% (95% CI, 12.03 - 28.25%), though prevalence was higher in men from low to medium income countries than men from high-income countries.

In the rating of risk factors for PAD, diabetes was rated second after smoking and a prevalence of 1.88% (95% CI, 1.60 - 2.14) of diabetes was noted in high-income countries versus a 1.47% (95% CI, 1.29 - 1.68) prevalence in low to medium income countries, and this is the income band for Zimbabwe as well (Human Development Indices and Indicators: 2018).

Chronically, the arterial walls will be gradually stenosed starting with small diameter arteries below the knees such is the case with early-stage PAD in asymptomatic diabetic patients (Sun et al., 2013; Peihua, 2003). However, lack of symptoms may not always be linked with early-stage PAD for evidence has indicated lack of symptoms in diabetic patients with late-stage PAD especially if they experience neuropathy or lead a sedentary lifestyle (Sun et al., 2013; Jude, 2004).

From the early asymptomatic stage, mild PAD then manifests as intermittent claudication, which is a pain in the calf which manifests on walking but is relieved by rest. The peripheral pulses will be mostly normal to mildly decrease while the skin of the lower legs and feet will still be normal. Mild intermittent claudication, in this case, occurs due to ischaemic pain in the leg musculature when the patients walk (Type 2 Diabetes in adults: management (NG28), NICE, 2015; Macleod et al., 2008).

1.1.3 Classification of PAD

Classification systems for PAD must be put in place to allow accurate diagnosis of its symptoms in each patient and this enables mapping how each patient will be treated. This consistent grading of patients will enable objective criteria of treating patients with a clinical follow up (Hardman et al., 2014). Prior evidence has indicated that several classification systems have been put in place for utilisation in the classification of PAD in clinical settings, direct patient management and research (Hardman et al., 2014; Rutherford et al., 1997). According to the classification by Rutherford et al., (1997), the asymptomatic grade zero (early-stage PAD) is the category where the patient will not be experiencing symptoms of claudication even though the detected asymptomatic PAD warrants early treatment to slow its progression into critical limb ischaemia.

The classification of PAD by Fontaine et al., (1954) was solely based on clinical symptoms without considering the use of other diagnostic tests, while the classification of PAD by Rutherford et al., (1997), resembles that of Fontaine et al., (1954) but with the addition of objective data in the form of non-invasive information from diagnostic tests, such as treadmill testing, six-minute walk, Ankle Brachial Index and pulse volume recordings (Hardman et al., 2014). Rutherford et al., (1997) also classified symptomatic PAD into acute and chronic forms and they advocated that each form requires a different treatment pathway (Hardman et al., 2014) and this showed a more focussed and effective management pathway for late-stage PAD.

Further classification of PAD by Rutherford et al., (1994) encompasses grade zero which is asymptomatic, then grades one, two and three where the grading of symptoms includes moderate to severe claudication, ischaemic rest pain, minor tissue loss and later major tissue loss. Systolic ankle blood pressure after exercise will be less than 50 mmHg in moderate to severe claudication while resting systolic ankle blood pressure in ischaemic rest pain symptoms will be less than 40 mmHg. However, in minor to major tissue loss, the systolic resting ankle blood pressure will be less than 60 mmHg (Hardman et al., 2014).

According to Rutherford et al., (1997), the asymptomatic category zero stage for early PAD would be confirmed in a patient who elicits the same pre- and post-ankle blood pressure after undergoing a treadmill exercise or reactive hyperaemia testing with thigh blood flow occlusion, while reduced post- ankle blood pressure is confirmed in patients with late-stage PAD (Hardman et al., 2014). Several prior studies have noted that, with moderate exercise, normal subjects maintain a stable ankle pressure or show a slight increase (Higashi et al., 2001; Philpott and Anderson, 2007) and this was partly owed due to the presence of normal bioavailability levels of nitric oxide and other vasodilatory metabolites in the endothelium of their arteries which affords adequate vasodilation to enable a compensatory increase in blood flow that occurs after this short period of tissue ischaemia (Higashi et al., 2001; Huang, 2005). However, this response is suppressed in patients with cardiovascular risk factors such as hypertension and diabetes, partly due to the presence of endothelial dysfunction in their arteries which may result in reduced bioavailability of nitric oxide and other vasodilatory metabolites (Higashi et al., 2001; Philpott and Anderson, 2007).

Diabetic patients with late-stage PAD thus experience claudication during exercise and physical activity as their arteries are not able to undergo the vasodilatory compensation to meet the enhanced demand for oxygen and metabolites. This as this can lead to further reductions in activity levels resulting in a progressive worsening of the symptoms associated with PAD from diabetes and a greater reliance on medication.

Peripheral Artery Disease is not preventable in cases such as increasing age (Kaku, 2010; Bhatia et al., 2004) and diabetes but its acceleration rate into critical limb ischaemia may be slowed down (Rutherford et al., 1997; Hardman et al., 2014).

1.1.4 Beetroot juice and therapeutic management of peripheral artery disease.

The UK and USA guidelines on adult diabetes management outline the prescription of Aspirin /Clopidogrel as antiplatelet therapy in patients with cardiovascular diseases, besides advising on smoking cessation, healthy eating of foods with high fibre, and foods with low glycaemic index sources of carbohydrate, increasing physical activity and exercise and self-monitored feet care (Eisenstein et al., 2017; Rooke et al., 2011, Hirsch et al., 2005; Type 2 Diabetes in adults: management (NG 28), NICE, 2015).

Diets containing natural inorganic nitrate are exogenous sources for the much-needed nitric oxide in patients suffering from highly inflammatory and oxidative diseases like Type 2 diabetes (Clements et al., 2014; Lundberg et al., 2008). Again, evidence has shown that these diets which are rich in inorganic nitrate are associated with inhibition of platelet aggregation, preservation and improvement of endothelial dysfunction which may be caused by diabetes in the arterial walls (Clements et al., 2014; Lundberg et al., 2008; Doel et al., 2005; Hyde et al., 2014). Some of the vegetable diets rich in natural inorganic nitrate include beetroot, green leafy vegetables such as spinach, rocket, Chinese cabbage and lettuce were also found to contain large sources of inorganic nitrate (Clements et al., 2014; Lundberg et al., 2008; Doel et al., 2005; Hyde et al., 2014). Prior evidence has indicated that that beetroot juice may improve blood flow via vasodilation in healthy participants resulting in improvement during exercise (Vanhatalo et al., 2011) and has been used successfully in the treatment and reduction of blood pressure in healthy participants (Webb et al., 2008; Hobbs et al., 2012) and subjects with cardiovascular disease and Type 2 Diabetes (Kenjale et al., 2011; Clifford et al., 2015; Siervo et al., 2013;

Bahadoran et al., 2015; Gilchrist et al., 2013) like participants who ingested dietary nitrate salts (Kapil, 2010; Bond et al., 2012).

Nitric oxide gas is produced endogenously from the amino acid L-arginine by three isoforms of nitric oxide synthases in the endothelium of blood vessels, and it is useful as an anti-oxidation defence system and an antiplatelet thus inhibiting the acceleration of atherosclerosis (Siervo et al., 2011; Steinberg, 2009, Steinberg and Wizturn, 2010 Kiboki, 2000). This evidence was discovered earlier by Cooke (1996), in his *in vivo* and *in vitro* studies with rabbits when high cholesterol chow was given to white rabbits for 10 weeks to induce atherogenesis and vascular disease in them which was noted in their thoracic arteries by 10 weeks as 30%-40% was involved in lesions and there was reduced NO activity in this state of their endothelium. Arginine was then added to 0.5% cholesterol diet of half the animals at 10, 14, 18 and 23 weeks as a way of inducing enhanced nitric oxide activity in the presence of pre-existing endothelial dysfunction and vascular disease. This administration of arginine restored nitric oxide activity in most of the rabbits at 14 and 18 weeks as evidenced by reduced thicknesses of lesions and plaque in the harvested thoracic aorta as compared to the prior thickness before arginine administration. This effect was associated with an apparent regression in atherogenesis leading to the conclusion that restoring nitric oxide activity reduced monocyte adhesion and accumulation in blood vessels (Cooke, 1996).

Evidence has shown that it is not easy to directly provide oral supplementation of nitric oxide or L-arginine to humans, but this can be done through consumption of dietary supplements (donor drugs) or vegetables rich in inorganic nitrate, like beets, celery, spinach, lettuce, radishes or cereals or cured meat thereby increasing the circulating nitric oxide independent of its endogenous nitric oxide synthases biosynthesis (Webb et al., 2008; Lundberg et al., 2008; Hord et al., 2009; Bahadoran et al., 2015; Clifford et al., 2015). Beetroot contains inorganic nitrate as the main bioactive component responsible for the reduction of blood pressure, endurance exercise interactions as well as cardiovascular interactions and in concurrence, studies which used beetroot with inorganic nitrate removed as a placebo intervention noted the improved blood flow via vasodilation and increased exercise endurance in the interventional groups (Vanhatalo et al., 2010; Bailey et al., 2009; Clifford et al., 2015).

Following oral consumption, nitrate is quickly absorbed in the stomach, duodenum and jejunum and availed in the circulation. It is later excreted from the circulatory system into the oral cavity where commensal bacteria anaerobes (via nitrate reductive enzymes) mainly found under the back of the tongue bio-activate nitrate and reduce it to nitrite in saliva (the entero-salivary circulation), while the larger portion of nitrate is excreted via kidneys (Kapil et al., 2010; Vanhatalo et al., 2010).

When this nitrite in the saliva is swallowed into the acidic stomach, some of it is bio-activated into nitric oxide then both the nitric oxide and nitrite are rapidly absorbed into the circulation peaking within 15 – 45 minutes after oral nitrate administration from nitrate salts but this bioavailability increases to 2.5 – 3 hours when the nitrite and nitric oxide will be availed from the entero-salivary circulation following ingestion of foods rich in inorganic nitrate like beetroot juice (Kapil et al., 2010; Vanhatalo et al., 2010; Webb et al., 2008). Accordingly, this evidence on the bioavailability of nitrite and nitric oxide within 2.5 – 3 hours was evidenced with a closely correlating reduction in blood pressure (Vanhatalo et al., 2010; Webb et al., 2008), with the increment of cyclic GMP (a sensitive marker for nitric oxide bioavailability (Kapil et al., 2010).

The main purpose of the availed nitric oxide is to maintain endothelial function in the inner walls of the arteries thus maintaining vascular homeostasis through maintaining the oxidative defence system, platelet function, vascular tone and the delicate balance between vasodilation and vasoconstriction (Clifford et al., 2015; Hobbs et al., 2012; Davignon and Ganz, 2004). Therefore this depletion in nitric oxide availability has been concluded as the main cause of endothelial dysfunction which is considered as a major risk factor for several cardiovascular disorders and in the pathogenesis of hypertension and atherosclerosis (Lidder et al., 2013; Joris and Mensik, 2013).

Beetroot juice is considered as a promising treatment in a range of clinical pathologies associated with oxidative stress and inflammation (Clifford et al., 2015; Bahadoran et al., 2015; Gilchrist et al., 2013). Being a source of inorganic nitrate, ingestion of beetroot juice increases the bioavailability of nitric oxide to manage these pathologies associated with diminished nitric oxide availability, such as diabetes, hypertension, dyslipidaemia to mention a few, thus diminishing the rate of atherosclerosis (Kapil, 2010; Clements et al., 2014; Clifford et al., 2015; Kannady et al., 2012). A study by Mcdonagh et al., (2018) showed that beetroot juice was one of the most effective dietary nitrate food forms which allowed effective nitrate metabolism and blood pressure reduction in normotensive adults.

Beetroot juice has been well researched and concentrations of about 5 mmol to 8 mmol and even more of natural inorganic nitrate in beetroot juice have been used in previous beetroot juice studies without any known adverse effects (Clifford et al., 2015; Gilchrist et al., 2013; Bahadoran et al., 2015; Kenjale et al., 2011, Webb et al., 2008, Vanhatalo et al., 2010), in other countries. To date, no serious adverse reactions were reported in prior studies of beetroot juice while the previously noted short term after-effects of oral beetroot juice intake include beeturia, red stools, reduction of blood pressure and mild gastrointestinal discomfort (Clifford et al., 2015; Gilchrist et al., 2013; Bahadoran et al., 2015; Kenjale et al., 2011; Vanhatalo et al., 2010; Webb et al., 2008).

This prior evidence on beetroot juice enabled the justification for the administering of beetroot juice to participants in the third investigation of this book and the sample for the beetroot juice which was administered to participants in the third investigation of this book is shown in figure 1.

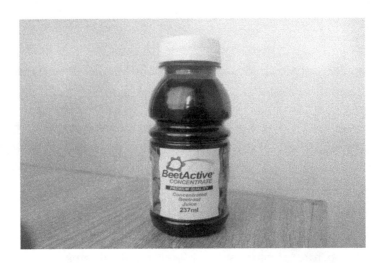

Figure 1 *Sample of beetroot juice which was administered to participants in the third investigation of this book.*

1.2 book Rationale

Previously, researchers have shown Ankle Brachial Index utilisation in improving accuracy for the prediction of cardiovascular risk and a low Ankle Brachial Index of less or equal to 0.90 has been associated with presence PAD (Rensick et al., 2004; Rooke et al., 2011; Sanna et al., 2011). Again prior evidence from the Preventive task Force did not support routine screening of asymptomatic individuals since this screening was deemed not to be able to detect the presence of peripheral artery disease (Rooke et al., 2011; Sanna et al., 2011). This, therefore, meant that an Ankle Brachial Index of greater or equal to 90 in asymptomatic individuals would not have mandated necessity of screening for PAD. However, it has also been noted that utilisation of Ankle Brachial Index only to quantify PAD had shortcomings since it is not able to provide the clinicians with objective data providing a clear picture of the clinical severity of the disease (Cacoub et al., 2009). On another note, prior studies have also shown that duplex ultrasound parameters (Rooke et al., 2011) such as peak systolic velocity (Randall et al., 2013) and pulsatility index (Campbell, 1986) were useful in detecting anatomic location and degree of stenosis of PAD. No prior evidence was found justifying the utilisation of ultrasound parameters to establish the effects of early-stage PAD in the lower limb blood flow of asymptomatic diabetic patients or non-diabetic participants at the point of writing up of this book. The second investigation of this book thus aimed to fill this literature gap by determining the effects of early-stage PAD on the lower limb blood flow of asymptomatic diabetic patients whose categorisation for early-stage PAD was confirmed with a normal reactive hyperaemia test (Rutherford et al., 1997; Hardman et al., 2014). The second investigation of this book utilised ultrasound parameters which came out as robust after being tested for repeatability in measuring lower limb blood flow in asymptomatic diabetic patients with early-stage PAD in the first investigation of this book.

By being diabetic asymptomatic patients already carry a risk factor for PAD and cardiovascular diseases (Sanna et al., 2011; Rooke et al., 2011) and early diagnosis would call for early introduction of interventional therapy. However, Rooke et al.,(2011) recommended antiplatelet therapy for individuals with asymptomatic lower extremity PAD to reduce the risk for cardiovascular diseases (Rooke et al.,2011) while UK NICE guidelines for type 2 diabetes management do prescribe Aspirin or Clopidogrel antiplatelet therapy only to patients with cardiovascular disease risk (Type 2 Diabetes in adults: Management (NG 28), NICE 2015).

On another note, prior evidence has shown that Aspirin or both Aspirin and Clopidogrel administration in both symptomatic and asymptomatic (early-stage PAD) patients as effective preventive antiplatelet therapy for cardiovascular disease such as myocardial infarction though they were associated with higher incidences of minor bleeding which were noted as higher in Aspirin therapy alone (Cacoub et al., 2009). The third investigation of this book was trying to fill this gap in the literature by aiming to establish blood flow effects which may occur after beetroot juice ingestion in the lower limb arteries of asymptomatic diabetic patients with early-stage PAD using ultrasound parameters. However, if the effects of beetroot juice ingestion on blood flow were to be significant and meaningful then this would be considered as therapeutic and beetroot juice ingestion may be an effective non-pharmacological alternative to improve blood flow and reduce blood pressure.

According to Sanna et al., (2011), current evidence on the epidemiology of PAD is confined to studies done in the Northern European and American countries and given the fact that epidemiology for atherosclerosis was found to be affected by factors such as genetics, diet, ethics, environment and lifestyle, it becomes possible that the findings for PAD in the southern countries of Europe and America may differ. These findings thus justify the undertaking of the second investigation of this book in utilising ultrasound parameters to detect the effects of early-stage PAD in the lower limb arterial blood flow of Zimbabwean Black/African diabetic patients. Again, to date, no such study has been undertaken in Zimbabwean Black/African diabetic patients.

The Zimbabwean Health Delivery System is experiencing the burden of many cardiovascular non-communicable diseases such as diabetes, stroke, heart attacks and chronic lung disease, and diabetes is a major contributor to deaths from cardiovascular diseases occupying the fourth place in the top ten (Hakim et al., 2005; Parirenyatwa and Gwinji, 2016-2020). Type 2 diabetes mellitus is one of the most prevalent chronic health conditions with an estimated 387 million people affected worldwide, (IDF, 2015) and Zimbabwe is one of the 32 African member countries of the International Diabetic Federation (IDF, 2015). The Zimbabwean country is equally battling with the chronic prevalence of Type 2 diabetes mellitus and its complications and the prevalence of Type 2 diabetes mellitus was 10%. The WHO estimated that 1% of total deaths in Zimbabwe were due to diabetes mellitus and in the year 2014, it was found amongst the national top 20 causes of mortality responsible for about 206 deaths (Parirenyatwa and Gwinji, 2016-2020). The number of new cases of diabetes mellitus in Zimbabwe for the age range of 0-24 years was 8

658 and for the age range of greater than 25 years, it was 102 077 (Parirenyatwa and Gwinji, 2016-2020).

The Zimbabwe National Health Strategy cost estimation for Non-Communicable Diseases which includes diabetes mellitus was projected to cost up to US$7.4bn from 2016 to 2020, while the mean per capita cost for these Non-Communicable Diseases was projected at US$ 91 (Parirenyatwa and Gwinji, 2016). Accordingly, the National Health Strategy for Zimbabwe (2016-2020) noted the shortage of basic commodities such as glucostrips and essential medicines and delayed utilisation of services as the major drawbacks to proper monitoring of diabetes mellitus and its complications in Zimbabwe. The report also noted that proper monitoring of diabetes mellitus in Zimbabwe was crucial to mitigate the rate of complications arising from poorly controlled blood glucose levels and this could be strengthened by promoting strategies seeking to address healthy life and diet, improvement of commodities availability and screening (Parirenyatwa and Gwinji, 2016 - 2020).

With this prior background on the Zimbabwean situation about diabetes mellitus, the third investigation of this book focussed on the ultrasound assessment of the acute effects of ingested beetroot juice on the lower limbs arterial blood flow of diabetic patients with early-stage PAD aiming to establish if the findings could contribute information towards an earlier and affordable non-pharmacological alternative for the management of blood flow and blood pressure in diabetic patients within the secondary healthcare set up of the Zimbabwean health delivery system. The background information on the Zimbabwean health delivery system indicated that ultrasound machines were available in secondary care district hospitals in Zimbabwe while beetroot is a readily available vegetable easily grown by Zimbabweans. See section 1.2.1 for more detail on the background of the Zimbabwean health delivery system.

Prior information from beetroot juice studies conducted in other populations has indicated multiple health benefits from ingestion of it such as reduction of blood pressure (Webb et al., 2008; Hobbs et al., 2012; Mcdonagh et al., 2018), the increment of time to exercise (Vanhatalo et al., 2011; Gilchrist et al., 2013) to mention a few and these changes in blood flow are hypothesised to result from vasodilation but to date, this has not been measured or reported.

1.2.1 Background information

In this book, the sample for diabetic patients with early-stage PAD was recruited from a quaternary care Hospital (Mpilo central hospital) diabetic clinic in the city of Bulawayo, Zimbabwe, while the sample for non-diabetic controls was recruited from the staff members and students of the National University of Science and Technology in the city of Bulawayo, Zimbabwe. Myself as the principal investigator for this book, am a lecturer in the department of Radiography formerly Applied Physics at the National University of Science and Technology in the same city of Bulawayo, Zimbabwe.

According to the most recent census carried out in Zimbabwe in 2012, the population of Zimbabwe is about 13 061 239 and the majority population is of the Black-African ethnic group (98.6%), while there is a minority population of Europeans (0.6%), Asians (0.2%) and mixed (0.4%) (Dzinotizei, 2013). The fact that Black/Africans formed the majority population in Zimbabwe and at the research centre made it possible to recruit the required sample size of diabetic patients from one homogenous ethnic group of Black/Africans for this book. Cacoub et al., (2009) noted that the epidemiology of PAD in various ethnic groups, various lifestyles and diets is not uniform, thus for this book it was important to recruit the required book sample size from a homogenous population.

Zimbabwe's health referral system is a four tiered-pyramidal system with the lower level primary health facilities (Clinics), secondary level facilities (District hospitals), tertiary level facilities (Provincial hospitals), and quaternary level facilities (Central hospitals), while the administrative activities and decision making in the public sector are governed by the Ministry of Health and Child

Care (Osika et al., 2010; Tapfumaneyi and Okello, 2014; Parirenyatwa and Gwinji, 2016). The healthcare facilities for Zimbabwe are also found in non-profit making facilities, church organisations, companies and profit-making private facilities. Primary care in Zimbabwe consists of clinics, polyclinics, private clinics, mission clinics, council municipal clinics and rural health centres. (Table 1). These are the first port of call health care centres for patients in both rural and urban centres and they are mostly manned by a group of nurses and nurse aides and the services provided include basic prevention, maternity and curative services (Osika et al., 2010; Tapfumaneyi and Okello, 2014; Parirenyatwa and Gwinji, 2016). Patients presenting with more serious symptoms beyond primary care health services are referred to district hospitals (Parirenyatwa and Gwinji, 2016).

Secondary care (district hospitals) in Zimbabwe receive referred patients from primary care facilities and these district hospitals represent the lowest care level manned by one or two medical doctors besides the registered general nurses, nurse aides, a radiographer/x-ray operator and other few healthcare professionals (Osika et al; 2010; Tapfumaneyi and Okello, 2014; Parirenyatwa and Gwinji, 2016).

District hospitals are equipped with basic radiology equipment which mostly includes an x-ray and an ultrasound machine, while missionary, private and company facilities are also able to serve as district hospitals and speciality issues which cannot be handled at the district level of care are referred to tertiary care (Osika et al; 2010; Tapfumaneyi and Okello, 2014). The fact that there are ultrasound machines in secondary care centres where primary care centres mostly refer their patients this means that would be feasible to implement the proposed findings of this book of screening for early-stage PAD in secondary care using duplex ultrasound. Enhanced early detection of PAD in diabetic patients whilst still in secondary care will prompt for early introduction of therapy which may be enhanced as ingestion of beetroot juice to maintain good blood flow and blood pressure, thus also reducing the numbers referrals congesting into tertiary and quaternary care centres as well.

Tertiary care consists of the provincial hospitals which are in eight out of ten provinces of Zimbabwe excluding Harare and Bulawayo provinces where quaternary care health facilities are found (Osika et al; 2010; Tapfumaneyi and Okello, 2014; Parirenyatwa and Gwinji, 2016). Various unique and difficult cases are referred from tertiary care hospitals in the provinces to the five central (quaternary care) hospitals, thus three in Harare, two in Bulawayo and one in Chitungwiza, and the most advanced equipment, staff and pharmaceuticals for dealing with the most severe cases are found in these quaternary care facilities. (Osika et al., 2010; Tapfumaneyi and Okello, 2014). More detail on the number of hospitals and primary healthcare centres in Zimbabwe is outlined in table 1.

Table 1 shows the profile of Zimbabwean healthcare facilities (Parirenyatwa and Gwinji, 2016).

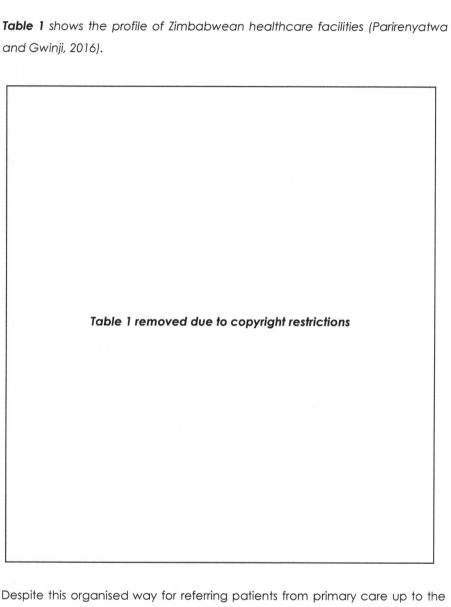

Table 1 removed due to copyright restrictions

Despite this organised way for referring patients from primary care up to the appropriate level of the healthcare in Zimbabwe, in the past ten years, this referral system stopped effectively working and lots of patients were now seeking primary or secondary care at all facility levels due to geographical convenience and this has led to overcrowding in tertiary and quaternary care hospitals (Parirenyatwa and Gwinji, 2016). This diabetic participant for this book was recruited carried out at a diabetic clinic for Mpilo central hospital, a quaternary care centre and its was feasible to recruit the required sample size of diabetic patients with early-stage (asymptomatic) PAD for this book due to this disorganised referral system which was apparent during the conduct of this book. However, in the 2016 - 2020 National Strategy of Zimbabwe, it was outlined that there was a need to enforce the initially existing referral system which was based on the primary health care approach and patient education to ensure that hospital services are only limited to those who need them thus reducing unnecessary overcrowding in the hospitals (Parirenyatwa and Gwinji 2016).

In the early 1990s to 2005, the Zimbabwean health delivery system was well funded and not very dependent on foreign donor funding, however since the depreciation of the economy from 2006-2008, the health system became underfunded and was heavily dependent on foreign donor funding (Osika et al., 2010; Tapfumaneyi and Okello, 2014; Parirenyatwa and Gwinji, 2016). The period of 2009-2012 saw the economy rebounding and beginning to reverse the consequences of the near-collapse of the health delivery system which occurred in 2008, although the period of 2013-2015 saw a dramatic drop in economic growth and the prospects for the next 5 years were predicted to remain sluggish (Tapfumaneyi and Okello, 2014; Parirenyatwa and Gwinji, 2016). However, as of the year 2016, all tertiary care hospitals in Zimbabwe are now equipped with computed tomography (CT) scanners, modernised ultrasound scanners and the modernised computed and digital radiography (CR and DR) X-ray machines, while quaternary care hospitals such as Mpilo and Parirenyatwa are now also having modernised Radiotherapy treatment machinery and Nuclear Medicine scanners, but Magnetic Resonance Imaging (MRI) is still currently available in private centres located in the Harare and Bulawayo provinces. In the National Health Strategy for Zimbabwe, 2016-2020, it was noted that there has been equitable commodities supply and security across referral levels particularly hospital levels (Parirenyatwa and Gwinji, 2016). This background information showed that despite the improved furnishing of tertiary and quaternary care centres with modernised equipment ideal for the care of the diabetic patients in late-stage PAD, there is the problem of flooding and overcrowding in these centres as well. Therefore, enhanced detection of early-stage PAD in asymptomatic diabetic patients with the readily available and cheap duplex ultrasound modality in secondary care centres will reduce overcrowding of tertiary and quaternary centres with diabetic patients having symptomatic PAD.

1.3 book aims and research questions

1.3.1 Introduction

The methodology of this book was conducted as three investigations which corresponded into each other and the first investigation is outlined in chapter 4, the second investigation is outlined in chapter 5 and finally, the third investigation is outlined in chapter 6. The aims and research questions for each of these three investigations are outlined accordingly in sections 1.3.2 to 1.3.4.1.

1.3.2 Investigation 1 aims

i) To determine the repeatability of ultrasound parameters in measuring blood flow in the diabetic lower limb arteries with early-stage PAD.

ii) To determine if there were any significant or meaningful differences in dependent variables (ultrasound blood flow parameters) between sessions.

1.3.2.1 Investigation 1 research questions

i) Can the ultrasound parameters repeatably measure blood flow in the diabetic lower limb arteries with early-stage PAD?

ii) Are there any significant or meaningful differences in dependent variables (ultrasound blood flow parameters) between sessions?

1.3.3 Investigation 2 aims

i) To compare blood flow between the diabetic lower limb arteries with early-stage PAD and non-diabetic controls using the ultrasound parameters.

ii) To determine if there were any significant or meaningful differences in dependent variables (ultrasound blood flow parameters) between groups.

1.3.3.1 Investigation 2 research questions

i) Is there a difference in blood flow between diabetic lower limb arteries with early-stage PAD and non-diabetic controls as determined by ultrasound parameters?

ii) Are the differences in, dependent variables between groups significantly meaningful?

1.3.4 Investigation 3 aim

To determine the acute effects of beetroot Juice ingestion on the diabetic lower limb arteries with early-stage PAD and non-diabetic controls using ultrasound parameters.

1.3.4.1 Investigation 3 research questions

i) Is there a change in blood flow within non-diabetic lower limb arteries after beetroot juice ingestion as determined by the ultrasound parameters (at 90 minutes; 150 minutes and 210 minutes)?

ii) Is there a change in blood flow within diabetic lower limb arteries after beetroot juice ingestion as determined by the ultrasound parameters (at 90 minutes; 150 minutes and 210 minutes)?

iii) Is there a difference in the blood flow changes between non-diabetic and diabetic lower limb arteries after beetroot juice ingestion as determined by the ultrasound parameters?

Chapter 2-Literature review

2.1 Introduction

The following chapter reviewed the literature on the diagnosis and therapeutic management of diabetes and PAD cited in this book. In this Narrative Critical Review (Demiris and Washington, 2019), the principal investigator utilised keywords extracted from the topic of each investigation as search items to extract relevant studies from the relevant journals in the Elsevier Science Direct, Pubmed, Scopus, Embase, Cochrane Library, PsycINFO, JAMA, JSTOR and CINAHL databases. The principal investigator then opened a desktop file and saved all these studies and then reviewed them against the research questions for each investigation accordingly. (See section 1.3.2.1 for the first investigation research questions; section 1.3.3.1 for the second investigation research questions and section 1.3.4.1 for the third investigation research questions). The studies were cited based on their clinical significance, the robustness of their methodology (where bias and error were minimised), internal validity and generalisability to the population under study (Umesh et al., 2016).

The principal investigator used the following keywords; *"Duplex ultrasound, repeatability, measurement error, peripheral artery disease, peak systolic velocity, pulsatility index, resistive index, vessel diameter"*, for the first investigation. For the second investigation, the principal investigator used the following keywords; *"peripheral artery disease, peak systolic velocity, pulsatility index, resistive index"*. Accordingly, for the third investigation, the principal investigator utilised the following keywords; *"peripheral artery disease, nitrite, nitric oxide, beetroot juice, blood pressure, peak systolic velocity"*. The principal investigator then summarised, synthesised and integrated the findings of these studies into the literature review of this book and referenced the articles which were incorporated in the write-up.

2.1.1 Methods for diagnosing PAD

Accurate diagnosis of PAD is crucial to allow timely specialist referral and improve patient outcome even when it can be an incidental finding in asymptomatic people attending a screening for other general examinations, (Rooke et al., 2011). Accordingly, the initial diagnosis for PAD with non-imaging tests is initially based on the eliciting of Intermittent claudication symptoms following graded treadmill testing, six-minute walks in the elderly patients, and abnormal reactive hyperaemic test or an Ankle Brachial Index of less or equal to 0.90 (Gerhard-Herman et al., 2016; Rooke et al., 2011; Norgren et al., 2007).

Early-stage/asymptomatic PAD categorised as Ankle Brachial Index greater or equal to 0.90, or normal reactive hyperaemic/ treadmill test was not recommended for screening with Ankle Brachial Index since the results from such patients were deemed not useful (Gerhard-Herman et al., 2016; Rooke et al., 2011) and duplex ultrasound was not recommended for the imaging of early-stage PAD in the current evidence during the writing up of this book. Prior evidence has advocated utilisation of duplex ultrasound in imaging late-stage (symptomatic) PAD as a modality to localise it and to map a way for surgical intervention, while a low Ankle Brachial Index of less or equal to 0.90 is significantly associated with classical cardiovascular risk factors (Sanna et al., 2011; Rooke et al., 2011). The sensitivity and specificity of duplex ultrasound (Collin et al., 2007; Leiner et al., 2005), as well as its reliability in the imaging of symptomatic (late-stage) PAD (Eiberg et al., 2010), has already been documented.

The available diagnostic imaging tests for symptomatic (late-stage) PAD besides duplex ultrasound include Magnetic Resonance Angiography, Computed Tomography Angiography and Digital Subtraction Angiography. However, duplex ultrasound and magnetic resonance angiography offer the least invasive options which avoid the use of ionising radiation and duplex ultrasound also offers the advantage of functional assessment of arterial stenosis. Though it is the most operator-dependent modality, Ultrasound is the cheapest and the most accessible imaging modality (Type 2 Diabetes in adults: management (NG 28), NICE, 2018; Macleod et al., 2008; Carthy, 2013; Eisenstein et al., 2017).

This book, therefore, aimed to fulfil the following gap in the literature as follows; i) determining the robustness of duplex ultrasound parameters in measuring blood flow in lower extremities of asymptomatic diabetic patients with early-stage PAD (first investigation)before utilising them with a larger sample size in the second and third investigations of this book.

ii) Determining the capability of robust ultrasound parameters from the first investigation in demonstrating the effects of early-stage PAD on the blood flow of asymptomatic diabetic patients (second investigation), and finally establishing the effects of beetroot juice ingestion on the lower limb blood flow of asymptomatic diabetic patients with early-stage PAD and non-diabetic controls who were imported from the second investigation, using robust ultrasound parameters from the first and second investigations alongside systolic blood pressure and diastolic blood pressure.

2.1.2 Treadmill testing and six-minute walks in diagnosing PAD

A standardised protocol for treadmill testing with or without Ankle Brachial Index assessments and the six minutes' walk has been recommended as class 1 level evidence in the ACC/AHA guidelines, (Hirsch et al., 2005; Rooke et al., 2011) to provide the most objective evidence of the magnitude of the functional limitation of claudication and to measure the response to therapy. A 6-minute walk test is an objective assessment of functional limitation of claudication and response to therapy in the elderly individuals and others not able to withstand treadmill testing (Hirsch et al., 2005; Rooke et al., 2011). Standardised exercise protocol on motorised Treadmill test are either grade or fixed to enable reproducibility of measurements in assessing the magnitude of functional limitation of claudication (Hirsch et al., 2005; Rooke et al., 2011). In this investigation, early-stage PAD was categorised according to the grade zero asymptomatic stage by Rutherford et al., (1997) and the objective assessment method was a normal reactive hyperaemic test.

2.1.3 Ankle Brachial Index in diagnosing PAD.

The diagnosis of symptomatic PAD has been exclusively achieved through the measurement of Ankle Brachial Index and according to Varaki et al., (2018); Rooke et al., (2011), Ankle Brachial Index is calculated by taking the higher of the systolic pressure of the dorsalis pedis or posterior tibial arteries and dividing it by the highest systolic brachial pressure. Therefore an Ankle Brachial Index greater than 1.0 and less or equal to 1.3 is considered normal, Ankle Brachial Index of less or equal to 0.90 is considered indicative of PAD and a risk for cardiovascular diseases, Ankle Brachial Index of 0.4 - 0.9 is indicative of intermittent claudication and Ankle Brachial Index of less than 0.4 indicates critical limb ischaemia (Gerhard- Herman et al., 2016). Prior evidence has again shown Ankle Brachial Index to be a highly sensitive and specific screening tool for PAD (Varaki et al., 2018; Rooke et al., 2011; Collins et al., 2007) and Ankle Brachial Index is a cheap and simple test which is also easily accessible to clinicians. However, Ankle Brachial Index has a weakness in that it does not provide objective data to assist the clinician with information about the severity of the disease.

A study by Sanna et al., (2011), examined the prevalence of asymptomatic PAD as determined by Ankle Brachial Index in Italian subjects presenting with moderate cardiovascular disease risk in the absence of diabetes or Overt vascular disease and their findings showed that a low Ankle Brachial Index of less or equal to 0.90 was associated with the presence of PAD in 22.9% of the sample of n = 5 112. Normal Ankle Brachial Index of 0.9 - 0.99 (23.9%) and greater than 0.99 (53.23%) was found in the rest of the sample participants. This study showed evidence that the Ankle Brachial Index could demonstrate low values of less or equal to 0.9 in asymptomatic patients with moderate cardiovascular disease risk in the absence of diabetes and overt vascular disease. Thus, the study concluded that such patients needed further screening for PAD. However, in the study by Sanna et al., (2011), Ankle Brachial Index could not demonstrate the presence of PAD in the remaining 87.13% of participants who had a normal value of greater or equal to 0.9. This remains a gap in the literature in this scenario where no other imaging modality has been recommended to rule out asymptomatic PAD in participants of a normal range Ankle Brachial Index of greater or equal to 0.90 during the writing up of this book. The second investigation of this book therefore aimed to provide some evidence to fill this gap in the literature by determining whether ultrasound parameters could demonstrate early-stage PAD in asymptomatic diabetic patients.

2.1.4 Colour Duplex Ultrasound for Imaging PAD

Colour duplex ultrasound combines the use of B-mode imaging/greyscale with the pulsed wave or continuous wave Doppler modes and colour when evaluating the anatomy and haemodynamic function of the vascular system (Varaki et al., 2018; Andersen, 2010). Thus, the B-mode images of arteries can be sampled for velocity spectra which are based on the Doppler principle when the ultrasound waveform undergoes frequency shift proportional to the velocity of the moving red blood cells in the arteries (Andersen, 2010; Hamments, 2014; Chavhan et al., 2008). This facility in colour duplex ultrasound enables haemodynamic changes in arteries due to PAD to be assessed through the utilisation of Doppler ultrasound parameters such as peak systolic velocity; resistive index and pulsatility index which are measured from the Doppler velocity spectrum waveform (Dhaliwal et al., 2007; Varaki et al., 2018; Hamments, 2014).

These Doppler ultrasound parameters undergo changes which correlate with the degree of stenosis caused by PAD in the arterial lumen. Therefore, the values of these parameters may be interpreted to confirm and grade late-stage (symptomatic) PAD (Andersen, 2010, Hodgkiss-Harlow and Bandyk, 2014; Hamments, 2014; Chavhan et al., 2008).

The B-mode/greyscale imaging enables the visualisation of two-dimensional images of arteries and information about diameter changes (Andersen, 2010; Varaki et al., 2018; Dhaliwal et al., 2007) due to PAD are seen. However, early detection of PAD in diabetic patients is highly recommended since it will enable therapeutic interventions to be initiated earlier in patients with a risk for cardiovascular diseases (Andersen 2010; Hernando and Conejero, 2007).

Prior evidence has shown that colour duplex ultrasound has documented high sensitivity (76%; 95% CI: 69% - 82%) and high specificity (93%; 95% CI: 91% - 95%) when compared with contrast-enhanced Magnetic Resonance Angiography with a higher sensitivity of about (84%; 95% CI: 78% - 89%) and specificity of about (97%; 95%: CI 95% - 98%) in detecting late-stage PAD in 295 referred patients (Leiner et al., 2005; Collins et al, 2007; Varaki et al., 2018). Again, colour duplex ultrasound is capable of demonstrating plaque which causes greater or equal to 50% arterial luminal reduction (Leiner et al., 2005; Varaki et al., 2018; Eiberg et al., 2010).

The reliability of colour duplex ultrasound in assessing blood flow in the lower limbs of diabetic patients with late-stage PAD was undertaken by Eiberg et al, (2010) in a prospective study of 530 participants and Digital Subtraction Angiography was the gold standard. In the study by Eiberg et al., (2010) colour duplex ultrasound was performed a day before the digital subtraction angiography examination for each patient over two years and the patients were suffering from intermittent claudication and critical limb ischaemia. The assessment was done in the common femoral arteries down to the pedal arteries in the worst symptomatic leg of each participant and the agreement between duplex ultrasound and digital subtraction angiography was obtained by using kappa. The study showed a very good agreement (k >0.8) or good agreement (0.8 ≥ k > 0.6) in most segments, but moderate agreement (0.6 ≥ k > 0.4) in the tibial-peroneal trunk and the peroneal artery. Agreement between colour duplex ultrasound and digital subtraction angiography was significantly higher (k = 0.75; 95% CI: 0.70 - 0.80) in the supra-genicular segments than in the infra-genicular segments (k = 0.63; 95% CI: 0.59 - 0.67) ($p < 0.001$) and again colour duplex ultrasound compared favourably with digital subtraction angiography in both tibial vessels and pedal arteries as well.

However, during the writing up of this book, there was no evidence regarding the utilisation of duplex ultrasound to quantify or screen for early-stage PAD in asymptomatic diabetic patients besides the recommendation of Ankle Brachial Index (Hirsh et al., 2005; Rooke et al., 2011). Despite its weakness in showing ballooned values of above 1.4 in calcified arteries of diabetic patients and elderly population (Chen et al., 2015), Ankle Brachial Index was shown weaker in showing normal values of 1-1.3 in participants who had asymptomatic PAD (Rensick et al., 2004). In earlier studies carried on participants with PAD, (Fowkes et al., 1991; Criqui et al., 1985; Hirsh et al., 2001; Dhaliwal 2007) it was noted that asymptomatic PAD was more common than symptomatic PAD in primary care settings despite a low awareness by physicians on this trend, and Hirsh et al., (2001) noted that under-diagnosis of PAD in primary care practice may be a barrier to effective secondary prevention of high ischaemic cardiovascular risk associated with PAD (Hirsh et al., 2001). Thus, Fowkes et al., (1991) and Criqui et al., (1985) in their studies recommended that there was a need for appropriate evaluation of individuals at high risk for cardiovascular diseases. The aim of the second investigation of this book was, trying to fill this gap in the literature by determining the capability of ultrasound parameters in demonstrating effects of early-stage PAD on the lower limb blood flow of diabetic patients, while Ankle Brachial Index was performed as a parallel test.

2.2 The ultrasound parameters.

The normal pulsed Doppler velocity spectra recorded from a peripheral lower extremity artery is triphasic with a narrow spectral range of velocities throughout the pulse cycle and this reflects that the arterial red blood cells are moving at a similar velocity and direction and the laminar flow pattern is not disturbed (Hodgkiss-Harlow and Bandyk, 2014). The velocity spectra waveform in each cardiac pulse for lower limb arteries reflects blood acceleration during systole, an early diastolic flow reversal caused by the propagated pressure pulse wave and its reflection from a higher downstream resistance followed by the late antegrade diastolic flow. The first component of systole results in measurements typically less than 125 cm/s for each arterial segment (Gerhard-Herman et al., 2006; Hodgkiss-Harlow and Bandyk, 2014). There is early diastolic flow reversal in the second wave of the waveform as left ventricular pressure reduces before aortic valve closure. However, in late diastole, there is a small amount of forwarding flow that reflects elastic recoil of vessel walls but this diastolic component is absent in stiff atherosclerotic vessels (Gerhard-Herman et al., 2006). A normal peripheral artery waveform is therefore characterised as high resistance and triphasic (Gerhard-Herman et al., 2006, Chavhan et al., 2008). See figure 2 for an illustration of normal triphasic waveforms in the common femoral artery, superficial femoral artery and popliteal artery.

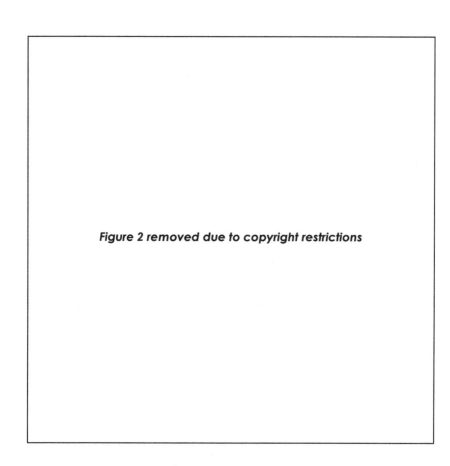

Figure 2 showing an illustration of normal triphasic flow in the common femoral artery, superficial femoral artery and popliteal artery as blood acceleration during systole, an early diastolic flow reversal and then a late antegrade diastolic flow (Cossman et al., 1989).

2.2.1 Peak systolic velocity

Peak systolic velocity is one of the most commonly used parameters in the grading of arterial stenosis, and its normal values in the tibial arteries of healthy subjects were about 55 ± 10 cm/s, and about 68 ± 14 cm/s in the popliteal arteries of healthy subjects (Hodgkiss-Harlow and Bandyk, 2014; Gerhard-Herman et al., 2006).

Peak systolic velocity has also been shown to be able to demonstrate PAD causing arterial luminal stenosis of greater or equal to 50% (Leiner et al., 2005; Eiberg et al., 2010; Franz et al., 2013; Gerhard-Herman et al., 2006). In another study by Yoshimura et al., (2006), it was shown that type 2 diabetic patients who developed cardiovascular complications on follow up had lower blood flow, *(p <0.01)*, which was due to increased vascular resistance, *(p <0.05)* and reduced peak systolic velocity caused by late-stage (symptomatic) PAD.

However, during the writing up of this book, no prior evidence was found in which peak systolic velocity was utilised to demonstrate haemodynamically - non-significant stenosis in asymptomatic diabetic patients with early-stage PAD and the aim of the second investigation of this book was to fill this gap in the literature by determining whether peak systolic velocity would be able to demonstrate effects of early-stage PAD in the popliteal artery, anterior tibial artery and posterior tibial artery of asymptomatic Black/ African diabetic patients. See figure 3 on how peak systolic velocity was measured in haemodynamically non-significant stenosis.

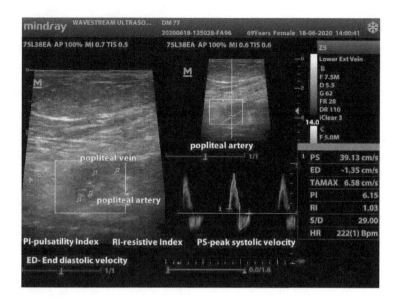

Figure 3 *showing manual trace measurement for peak systolic velocity (39.13 cm/s), end-diastolic velocity (-1.35 cm/s), resistive index (1.03) and pulsatility index (6.15 cm/s) in a haemodynamically - non-significant stenosis in the popliteal artery by the principal investigator.*

2.2.2 Pulsatility index

Pulsatility index is defined as the ratio of the peak to the peak height of the Doppler waveform to the mean height. Pulsatility index together with resistive index provide information about blood flow and resistance which cannot be obtained from measurements of peak systolic velocity, and it is calculated from the following formula in equation 1;

$$\text{Pulsatility index} = \frac{\text{Peak systolic velocity} - \text{End Diastolic Velocity}}{\text{Mean Velocity}} \qquad 1$$

Prior evidence (Hodgkiss–Harlow and Bandyk 2014; Harrington, 2012) has indicated that normal pulsatility index values in the lower limb arteries for healthy subjects should be greater than 4 while values of less or equal to 4 reflect proximal in-flow occlusive disease. In the common femoral arteries and popliteal arteries, pulsatility index values for healthy individuals are greater than 6 and greater than 8 respectively (Hodgkiss–Harlow and Bandyk 2014; Harrington, 2012). When there is increased resistance to blood flow, the peak systolic velocity peak tends to lower down and the end-diastolic velocity will be reduced or even absent, thus from equation 1 one above, the value of pulsatility index, in this case, will accordingly get reduced. This means that both the peak systolic velocity values and accordingly pulsatility index values can be used to demonstrate changes in blood flow due to PAD. However, during the writing of this book, no evidence was found which utilised pulsatility index in the to demonstrate effects of PAD in the lower limbs of asymptomatic diabetic patients with early-stage PAD and the aim of this book was to partly fill this gap in evidence by utilising pulsatility index to assess effects of early-stage PAD in the blood flow of the popliteal arteries, posterior tibial arteries and anterior tibial arteries of asymptomatic Zimbabwean Black/African diabetic patients.

2.2.3 Vessel diameter inner to inner

Vessel lumen radius has a profound effect on the volume of flow and according to Poiseuille's law the primary factors affecting resistance to flow are the radius of the vessel lumen, length of the vessel and the viscosity of blood as shown in equation 2;

$$\text{Flow volume} = \frac{\text{pressure gradient} \times \text{radius of the vessel}^4}{\text{length of vessel} \times \text{viscosity of blood}} \qquad 2$$

Accordingly, a decrease in vessel radius increases the resistance to blood flow to the 4th power, but in large parallel arteries, a stenotic lesion will have haemodynamic effects when the arterial radius would have been reduced by 60%, and while for, any given radius reduction the longitudinal pressure drop along the length of the lesion will be significantly enhanced by the presence of turbulence (Harrington, 2012; Hodgkiss-Harlow and Bandyk, 2014). Prior evidence has indicated the normal lumen diameter of popliteal arteries of healthy subjects as 0.5 cm ± 0.1 and for tibial arteries as 0.3 cm ± 0.4 (Hodgkiss-Harlow and Bandyk, 2014), thus in the studied population's vessel diameter values less than the indicated normal values will be indicative of PAD. Sanna et al., (2011) indicated that the epidemiology for atherosclerosis may be affected by factors such as genetics, ethnicities, diet and lifestyle, this means the findings of this book on vessel lumen diameter of Black/Africans were bound to be different from the published dimensions of the European countries.

2.2.4 Resistive Index

Blood flows from a region of high pressure to a low-pressure region because of an existing pressure gradient. Blood does encounter resistance to its flow and will only flow if the pressure gradient exceeds resistance and this is illustrated in the Bernoulli equation (Alexander, 2017) as follows in equation 3.

$$\text{Flow volume} = \frac{Pressure\ gradient}{Resistance} \qquad 3$$

During systole, the blood pressure will be from the contracting heart while during diastole the blood pressure will be from the elastic recoil of large arteries. The systolic pump is stronger and moves blood forward even if the downstream resistance is very high, but the diastolic pump is weaker and is affected by downward resistance such that there will be reduced or no forward diastolic flow with increasing resistance. The resistive index is calculated from the following formula in equation 4.

$$\text{Resistive Index} = \frac{\text{Peak systolic velocity} - \text{End diastolic velocity}}{\text{Peak systolic velocity}} \qquad 4$$

However, since there was no prior evidence on the utilisation of resistive index to demonstrate the effects of PAD in the lower limb arteries blood flow of asymptomatic diabetic patients with early-stage PAD, this book aimed to provide evidence for filling this gap in the literature.

2.3 Contribution to the knowledge

The contribution to knowledge from the first investigation of this book is evidence on the robustness of ultrasound parameters in measuring blood flow in the lower limbs of asymptomatic Zimbabwean Black/African diabetic patients with early-stage PAD. The second investigation of this book contributes evidence on the capability of ultrasound parameters in demonstrating the effects of early-stage PAD on the lower limb blood of asymptomatic Zimbabwean Black/African diabetic patients.

The third investigation of this book contributes evidence on the effects of beetroot juice ingestion on the lower limb blood of asymptomatic Zimbabwean Black/African diabetic patients with early-stage PAD and non-diabetic controls as determined by the ultrasound parameters, systolic blood pressure and diastolic blood pressure. The ultrasound parameters which were combined as a diagnostic protocol in this book have been widely used in studies which undertook colour duplex ultrasound assessments of lower limb arteries for late-stage PAD (Leiner et al., 2005; Eiberg et al., 2010; Franz et al., 2013; Kapil et al., 2010), though this is the first time that the ultrasound parameters which include peak systolic velocity, pulsatility index resistive index and vessel diameter inner to inner have been combined this way.

Chapter 3-book methodology

3.1 Overview of experimental research investigations

This book was conducted as three investigations which corresponded into one another. The first investigation is outlined in chapter 4, the second investigation is outlined in chapter 5 while the third investigation is outlined in chapter 6. This chapter outlines the main methodological steps which were undertaken in all the three investigations overall. See section 3.2 for the summarised book methodology flow diagram. However, specific methodological steps for each investigation are also outlined in each of the three chapters separately. The principal investigator who undertook this book data collection and statistical analysis was me. I am a practising Sonographer and a diagnostic radiographer (Appendices N1, N2 and L) with my private ultrasound rooms (Appendices Q1 to Q4) in the city of Bulawayo, Zimbabwe and I hold certificates in Diagnostic Medical Ultrasound training from the Burwin Institute of Canada (2011-2012) (Appendix I, J, and K) as well as local accreditation by the Zimbabwe Allied Health Practitioners' council (appendices N1 and N2). I also hold a Diploma in Diagnostic Radiography from the University of Zimbabwe, School of Radiography, Harare (2000), A Master's Degree in Professional Development studies (health and Social care) from the University of Salford (2009) and I am a current Radiography lecturer in the Department of Radiography, formerly the Department of Applied Physics at the National University of Science and Technology in Bulawayo, Zimbabwe. I also hold a prior in-house training experience in vascular ultrasound of more than 10 years.

I underwent mentorship by a Bulawayo based Specialist Radiologist in colour Doppler ultrasound mapping in 2015 after enrolling for my PhD studies with the University of Salford in November 2014. See the acknowledgements section for more detail of the mentorship done.

During the conduct of all the three experimental investigations for this book, I had the diabetic clinic physician on the cover to monitor the participants for any unexpected reactions during the conduct of the book. The diabetic clinic-based physician on the cover also undertook the reactive hyperaemic tests in the presence of the principal investigator in the diabetic clinic during the recruitment stages which enabled the screening of the patients into the early-stage PAD category.

The ultrasound measurements and Ankle Brachial Index measurements for this book were undertaken by me in my private ultrasound rooms in the city of

Bulawayo (suite 302A, 3rd-floor Halyet house, corner Josiah Tongogara street and 9th avenue) (appendices Q1 to Q4), The laboratory for blood testing was also situated at the same premises as my private ultrasound rooms in 4th floor (appendix E5). The recruited patients were given money for bus fare to travel to the private ultrasound rooms in town for blood testing and ultrasound measurements son their specific booked dates which were set by the research assistants during recruitment in the diabetic clinic (Appendix V2).

The two research assistants who recruited participants were nurse aides who worked for my private ultrasound rooms and they also underwent prior training by me on how to undertake the socio-medical history of the participants, recruitment of participants and follow up with bookings, collation of data on Microsoft excel sheets, participants' preparation before blood tests and ultrasound measurements and finally aftercare of the participants.

The ultrasound machine and blood pressure machine used for this book belong to my private ultrasound rooms and quality control testing was done by my local PhD adviser who is a Medical physicist by profession using a Brachytherapy. Quality Assurance Phantom (model 045). See appendix W for more detail on this phantom.

The funding for this book was done by the Research board grant from the National University of Science and Technology, Zimbabwe (appendices V1 and V2) and Beetroot juice was imported from Neal's Yard Health shop based in South African (Appendix T). The ethical process was approved by the Medical Research Council of Zimbabwe (appendices O and U) and the Salford University ethics committee (Appendix S).

3.2 book Methodology Flow diagram

Investigation 1

> Repeatability study which aimed to establish the within sessions and between sessions reliability and measurement error magnitude of ultrasound parameters consisting of peak systolic velocity, pulsatility index, resistive index and vessel diameter inner to inner in measuring lower limb blood flow in the lower limb arteries of a cohort of asymptomatic Zimbabwean Black/African diabetic patients with early-stage PAD.

Decision making 1
Dorsalis pedis artery measurements dropped in both groups due to inconsistent vessel diameter inner to inner measurements. Vessel diameter was then excluded from further analysis in the second and third investigations due to increased measurement errors in the posterior tibial artery.

Investigation 2

> Comparative cohort study aiming to determine capability of robust parameters from first investigation in demonstrating the effects of early stage PAD on lower limb arteries blood flow of Zimbabwean Black/African diabetic patients through comparison with non - diabetic controls. This stage also aimed to establish any significant or meaningful differences in dependent variables between the two groups which were in comparable conditions.

Within sessions, reliability was essential in this investigation since it had only been established in diabetic patients during the first investigation but not yet in the non-diabetic controls in this investigation. Therefore, this was done to allow comparison to be done between groups.

Decision making 2
Pulsatility index was concluded as not robust in demonstrating effects early-stage PAD in the blood flow of the anterior tibial arteries and posterior tibial arteries.
The resistive index was dropped to enable a more focused assessment of peak systolic velocity alongside systolic blood pressure and diastolic blood pressure on the popliteal arteries blood flow during the third investigation.

Investigation 3

> Prospective quasi-experimental study aimed at determining if consumption of beetroot juice resulted in meaningful changes in lower limb arterial blood flow in the two groups and if the magnitude of any changes in blood flow after beetroot juice ingestion were greater in one group compared to the other as determined by robust ultrasound parameters from the second investigation alongside systolic blood pressure and diastolic blood pressure.

Decision making 3
Only the popliteal arteries were assessed for blood flow changes after beetroot juice intake utilising peak systolic velocity alongside systolic blood pressure and diastolic blood pressure in both groups to minimise the error of measurements due to timing since blood flow changes quickly wan away.
The resistive index will be assessed alongside peak systolic velocity in the longitudinal study for post-doctoral work to establish long term effects of beetroot juice ingestion.
Between sessions, repeatability during the first investigation was essential to enable determining measurement error across different sessions for the intervention of beetroot juice during the third investigation as it was essential to determine if any changes were greater than the associated measurement error of the assessment method.

3.3 book experimental design

The first investigation for this book was a repeatability study, and the aim was to quantify both within sessions and between sessions reliability and measurement error of ultrasound parameters (dependent variables) in measuring blood flow in the lower limb arteries of a cohort of 10 Black/African diabetic patients with early-stage PAD to establish the robustness of the measurement method before its utilisation in gathering data for the bigger sample participants in the second and third investigations. The principal investigator adopted a within-subjects and between sessions repeated measures design to establish within-session and between-session reliability and measurement error of ultrasound parameters in measuring blood flow in the popliteal arteries, anterior tibial arteries, posterior tibial arteries and dorsalis pedis arteries. The principal investigator then imported the emerging robust ultrasound parameters from the first investigation for further analysis into the second investigation.

During the conduct of the first investigation, the principal investigator put measures and controls in place in the inclusion and exclusion criteria and the methodology to minimise bias such that the ultrasound parameter measurements which were made on the same subject depended on the within-subject standard deviations which were quantified as the measurement errors. The second aim of the first investigation was to establish if there were any significant or meaningful changes in dependent variables (ultrasound blood flow parameters) between sessions.

The second investigation of this book was a comparative cohort study and the aim was to determine the capability of the robust ultrasound parameters from the first investigation in demonstrating early-stage PAD on the blood flow of the popliteal arteries, anterior tibial arteries, and posterior tibial arteries of 35 Black/African asymptomatic diabetic patients through comparison with 36 non-diabetic controls while the two groups were in comparable conditions.

The principal investigator allowed recruitment of the 10 diabetic patients from the first investigation into the second investigation of 35 diabetic patients. The principal investigator adopted a within-subjects repeated measures design to determine the within-session reliability of ultrasound parameters (dependent variables) to enable comparison between groups. Within-sessions, reliability was essential in this investigation since the principal investigator had established reliability only in the diabetic patients during the first investigation but not yet in the non-diabetic controls the second investigation. The principal investigator performed the ultrasound measurements in a cohort of Black-African participants in the age range of 18 - 70 years for both groups and those parameters which came out showing a significant difference between the two groups were interpreted as those able to demonstrate the outcome of early-stage PAD on lower limb blood flow and these were imported into the third investigation.

The third investigation of this book was a prospective quasi-experimental study and the aim was to determine if consumption of beetroot juice could result in meaningful changes in lower limb blood flow both within and between the two groups of participants imported from the second investigation using ultrasound parameters and blood pressure. Secondly, the third investigation aimed to identify the magnitude of any changes in blood flow after beetroot juice ingestion between individual time points within and between groups and also between the two groups across four-time points using ultrasound parameters and blood pressure.

The principal investigator adopted a within and between subjects repeated measures design to determine changes in the dependent variables both within and between groups respectively. Between-sessions reliability which was performed by the principal investigator in the second investigation was essential to enable the determining of measurement error across different sessions for the intervention of beetroot juice in the third investigation. This was essential since the principal investigator needed to determine if any changes were greater than the associated measurement error of the assessment method.

This book design was rigorous since all in the three investigations, the principal investigator gathered the data prospectively such that the outcomes were unknown to her at the time of participants' enrollment. The principal investigator put the following measures and controls in place to minimise of bias and to increase the rigour of the book methodology;

i) A strict inclusion and exclusion criteria for participants.

ii) Establishment of the robustness of the measurement method before larger sample measurements.

iii) Diet preparations by patients before measurements.

iv) Prior relevant experience in vascular imaging by the principal investigator.
v) Prior training of research assistants.

vi) Blinding of the principal investigator.

vii) Simple random sampling during participants' recruitment.

See sections 3.6 and 3.4 for more detail on the detail of the measures and controls which were put in place during the conduct of the three investigations.

3.4 book inclusion and exclusion criteria

The participants for this book were recruited by the trained research assistants from the Black-African ethnic group which made the majority population (98.6%) understudy at both research sites, thus it was feasible for them to obtain sample sizes which had been predetermined by the principal investigator. See section 3.5 on the recruitment plan for more detail. A homogenous Zimbabwean Black/African population enabled the eradication of the potential counteracting variables which could have emanated from a sample of participants from different ethnic groups.

Mpilo Central hospital is a quaternary care centre in the Zimbabwean health delivery system and inside the diabetic clinic, there were many patients in various stages of PAD. This was so because in the past 10 years the initially existing referral system stopped working effectively such that patients were now seeking for any level of care (primary or secondary) at all health facility levels due to geographic convenience (Osika et al, 2010; Tapfumaneyi and Okello, 2014; National Health Strategy for Zimbabwe, 2007 – 2013).

The principal investigator put a control for the age limit for the recruited adult participants at 18 - 70 years, since the consenting age for adults in Zimbabwe is 18 years and also the fact that type 2 diabetes usually starts manifesting from adolescence onwards (Kaku, 2010; Bhatia et al., 2014). However, the age of the recruited participants was limited up to 70 years since there is evidence that there is an increased risk of late-stage PAD in subjects of 70 years and above (Macleod et al., 2008; Type 2 Diabetes in adults management (NG 28) NICE, 2015; Klabunde, 2007; Hernando and Conejero, 2007) such that the probability of getting a sample of participants with early-stage PAD in this category was low.

The principal investigator again put a measure to exclude pregnant participants from all the three stages of this book because prior evidence has shown that blood pressure decreases while systemic blood flow increases as a result of systemic vasodilation in pregnancy (Mahendru et al., 2014; Sanghavi and Rutherford, 2014), therefore there were bound to be inconsistencies in blood flow if the lower limbs of pregnant participants were to be measured together with non-pregnant participants. This exclusion resulted in minimisation of measurement error which could have emanated from inconsistent basal blood flow in the participants before the undertaking of the measurements. In this book, therefore, all the patients of the childbearing age who were unsure of their last menstrual dates were excluded from the book.

A measure to exclude smokers and ex-smokers from the book was put in place by the principal investigator because there is a strong correlation between tobacco smoking and PAD (Hernarndo and Conejero, 2007; Klabunde, 2007), therefore it would not have been possible to get a representative sample of diabetic subjects with early-stage PAD amongst smokers and ex-smokers (Klabunde, 2007; Hernando and Conejero, 2007). This was done to reduce bias from the misclassification of exposure and outcomes which would have emanated if participants of different stages of PAD were to be recruited.

During the conduct of the three investigations of this book methodology, the research assistants utilised non-probability Convenience sampling (Glen, 2015) put in place by the principal investigator when recruiting participants for this book. Despite the disadvantage of inability to generalise study results to a wider population through convenience sampling (Glen, 2015), in this book, this sampling method appeared the most ideal one for recruiting the required sample of participants with the limited resources and budget which was allotted to it. The limited resources for this book again made it impossible to reach every member of the population of diabetic patients at Mpilo central hospital to afford them an equal chance at being selected. Again, this sampling method had a weakness of introducing selection bias of diabetic participants since the participants selected were those who were available at the diabetic clinic when recruitment was being carried out. Both groups of participants for this book were drawn from the same Zimbabwean Black/African population which was easily accessible during the gathering of data and there is a noted higher incidence of diabetes and its complications in this type of population (Parirenyatwa and Gwinji, 2016-2020).

3.5 book recruitment strategy

The recruitment of participants in this book was voluntary and participants were allowed to drop out anytime during the study if they so wished without them being inconvenienced in any way. A lapse time of at least twenty-four hours was allowed so that the participants could decide whether to participate or not. If willing to participate, the participants were to confirm by signing the consent forms, and this was stressed in the information sheets.

Diabetic patients with early-stage PAD for the first and second investigations of this book were recruited by the research assistants as they came to Mpilo central hospital's diabetic clinic during the weekdays when the clinic was open thus, from Tuesday to Thursday and permission had been granted by Mpilo central hospital board of ethics to allow this book to be carried out at their institute. The fact that this central hospital had a larger population of the Black-African patients with type 2 diabetes with the various stages of PAD, it became possible for the research assistants to recruit the required sample sizes which had been predetermined by the principal investigator. The principal investigator set the priority alpha at $p \leq 0.05$ and the required sample size for the first investigation was 10 diabetic patients with early-stage PAD and for the second investigation, it was 71 participants consisting of one group of 35 diabetic patients with early-stage PAD and the second group of 36 non-diabetic controls and these two groups from the second investigation were later imported into the third investigation.

As each of the asymptomatic diabetic patients entered the physician's room for their usual consultation, the attending physician undertook the reactive hyperaemic test in the presence of the principal investigator and then indicated on the recruitment form if the patient was eligible to be categorised as having early-stage PAD. The form was then handed over to research assistants waiting outside, who upon checking the forms would recruit all ticked participants with early-stage PAD. The right leg for each diabetic participant was recruited into the sample for the sake of consistency thus thirty-five legs were recruited.

Accordingly, the sample for the non-diabetic control group was feasibly recruited from the National University of Science and Technology volunteering staff and students through a mass advert which was designed by the principal investigator and sent to the mass email for the University staff and students. The two research assistants then recruited the volunteering staff and students who responded to the advert until a sample size of 36 -non-diabetic controls which had been predetermined by the principal investigator was achieved for the second investigation.

The research assistants utilised the Qdiabetes risk calculator (2015) to screen for the non-diabetic control group participants. Recruitment for participation in this control group was similarly voluntary just as was outlined for the diabetic participants and this was stressed in the advert which was a flight on the mass students' and staff members' website. The justification for having the National University of Science and Technology, Zimbabwe as the recruitment place for control group participants was because the place was close and convenient to the principal investigator researcher and to other institutes where the research was being carried out. The right leg for each participant in the control group was similarly recruited for the sake of consistency and 36 legs were recruited.

3.6 Patient preparation for all investigations

Demographic data such as the socio-medical history of participants were gathered by the two research assistants using a validated Qdiabetes risk calculator. The research assistants simply asked the patients to tick boxes of the required information on the information sheets which had a language of their choice amongst the three main languages spoken in Zimbabwe which include English, Shona and Ndebele. The research assistants were not medical professionals themselves but nurse aides. See section 3.2 for more detail on the research assistants. This measure minimised recall bias during the collection of socio-medical history since the research assistants were unfamiliar with the exposures and outcomes of this book.

The two research assistants instructed the diabetic patients to adopt a low nitrate vegetable diet and no meat or fish for three days before testing and they were told to fast six to twelve hours before the examination.

The research assistants instructed the patients to avoid alcohol at least forty-eight hours before the examination which was booked at eight o'clock in the morning at the diabetic clinic and the patients were advised not to take their prescribed diabetic and high blood pressure medications but to bring them on their appointment day. The justification why the principal investigator instructed the diabetic patients to avoid taking their medications in the morning was because the patients were made to fast 6 hours before undertaking blood flow and blood pressure measurements, thus they had a high chance of sliding into hypoglycaemia. However, the principal investigator later instructed diabetic patients to take their medications during the third investigation while ingesting beetroot juice to enable them to metabolise the small number of carbohydrates in the ingested beetroot juice and avoid destabilising their blood sugar levels.

Again the principal investigator later allowed the participants to take their blood pressure reducing medications after completing the third investigation after 210 minutes of ingesting beetroot juice. See section 6.4.2 in chapter 6 for more detail on this justification.

All these preparation measures were put in place by the principal investigator to minimise the effects of a nitrate-rich diet, a recent meal, alcohol and medication on the basal blood flow of the participants before the undertaking of blood flow measurements to reduce measurement error (all investigations) as well as avoiding the masking of the true effects of beetroot juice on blood flow (third investigation).

To check on compliance to prior preparation instructions by the participants the research assistants instructed the participants to diarise all the foods they had eaten three days before the undertaking of measurements and this enabled them to rebook participants who had failed to comply with prior dietary preparations.

All the control settings listed above-enabled minimisation of measurement error since in all the three investigations, participants needed to have a constant basal blood flow which was not influenced by the external factors controlled above. These measures then allowed the effects of early-stage PAD on blood flow during the first and second investigations, and the effects of beetroot juice intake on blood flow during the third investigation to be assessed with the reduced measurement error.

The research assistants gave the participants a refreshment of 100% fruit juice and a low sugar biscuit after completing the first investigation and also after completing the third investigation then allowed the participants to take their prescribed diabetic and blood pressure reducing medications (end of the first investigation, section 4.4.3) and their blood pressure reducing medications (third investigation, section 6.4.2). The principal investigator observed the participants for about 20 minutes before dismissing them to go home.

3.7 Body Mass Index and Ankle Brachial Index measurements

The two research assistants measured and recorded the participants' weight and height and collated these findings on Microsoft excel sheets with anonymised codes assigned to each participant alongside the socio-medical history of each patient. The principal investigator later calculated Body Mass Index values for each anonymously coded patient using equation 5 as follows;

$$Body\ Mass\ Index = \frac{weight}{height^2} \qquad 5$$

See appendix D which was used to collect data for Body Mass Index and Appendix F for the collated demographic raw data.

The principal investigator calculated Body Mass Index for the participants to enable documentation of their health status by measuring their body fat. However, Bell et al., (2018) showed that body mass index is not an accurate measure of total body fat since it does not distinguish fat from muscle or locate where the stored fat is in the body. Despite this weakness Body Mass Index was utilised to establish the general health status of participants in this book since the limitations of body mass index are mostly associated with athletic populations (Mitchell et al., 2014; Dickerson et al., 2011).

The supplying company representative for the automated blood pressure machine (*CareVue, Shenzhen, China*) performed calibration on it as per the manufacturer's specifications during commissioning before it was utilised by the principal investigator in this book for measuring Ankle Brachial Index and Blood pressure. See Figure 4 for more detail. The company representative inducted the principal investigator on how to carry out basic quality control tests for the blood pressure machine were as follows;

i) Wiping the monitor weekly to remove dust and debris.

ii) Checking and cleaning the filter weekly to remove dust and other particles (www. heartland medical.com).

The principal investigator performed Ankle Brachial Index for the two groups of participants after a supine rest of about 10 minutes and recorded the highest ipsilateral ankle pressure and subsequently divided it by the highest ipsilateral upper arm pressure. The principal investigator calculated the Ankle Brachial Index values for each participant which were then collated in Microsoft excel sheets with anonymised identification codes for each participant by the research assistants. See figure 4 for an illustration showing the measurement of blood pressure. In this book, the principal investigator performed the Ankle Brachial Index as, a parallel test to the ultrasound parameters' measurements. The upper arms and ankles blood pressure measurements were taken at a similar site on each participant.

The principal investigation performed Ankle Brachial Index measurements on the day of the ultrasound booking soon after the undertaking of blood tests in the laboratory which was located upstairs from the ultrasound private rooms. Blood tests to determine glycaemic control and renal function were important to establish the general health of the participants.

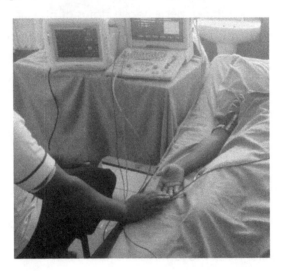

Figure 4 *Principal Investigator measuring Blood pressure on the right upper arm with an automated blood pressure machine (CareVue, Shenzhen China). This was performed on both upper arms and both ankles of each participant (Current book).*

3.8 Duplex Ultrasound parameters measurements

Qualitative assessment of the ultrasound scanner was done, (Goodsitt et al., 1988; Russel, 2014), before the assessment of the ultrasound parameters for repeatability. These qualitative assessments were done by a "Medical Physicist," using a Brachytherapy Quality Assurance (QA) phantom (Model 045, Universal Medical Inc. Norwood, MA, USA) which was utilised to perform a quality assessment of the ultrasound scanner for this book. See appendix W for more detail. Though originally designed for trans-rectal ultrasound QA and calibration of brachytherapy systems, in this book the phantom was utilised to test the 7.5 – 10.0 MHz probe to perform the following;

i) Internal grid assessment for testing lateral resolution and the axial resolution was done and the error margin after three trial measurements was 3% and 2% respectively reflecting the good performance of the ultrasound scanner. This quality control check for axial and lateral resolution (Goodsitt et al., 1988; Russel, 2014) was performed to reduce the error from measurements which could result from poor quality of ultrasound images which could have compromised the measurements for the three investigations.

The other basic quality control tests carried on the ultrasound scanner by the PhD advisor included physical and mechanical inspection, display monitor fidelity and image uniformity and the justification for carrying out this procedure was to reduce error in the ultrasound parameters measurements which could be due to a faulty scanner as well as prevention of any chances infection or electrical fault hazards (Goodsitt et al., 1988; Russel, 2014) affecting the participants during the study.

The ultrasound parameters measurements were similarly performed during the conduct of the three investigations by the principal investigator. However, specific modifications undertaken for each investigation stage are outlined within the methodology section of each investigation separately. The principal investigator performed ultrasound parameters measurements which included pulsatility index, peak systolic velocity, resistive index, vessel diameter inner to inner from an ultrasound machine (Mindray model Z5, Shenzhen, China) with a linear array probe which had a variable frequency of 7.5 – 10.0 MHz. The linear array probe utilised by the principal investigator has short wavelengths but high frequency which enabled high-resolution images during scanning for superficial structures like blood vessels (Hamments, 2014; Hwang, 2017). This justification was deducted from the wave equation (Hamments, 2014, Hwang,

2017) which relates wavelength to the speed and frequency of the ultrasound wave as follows in equation 6;

$$ultrasound\ beam\ wavelength = \frac{Speed\ of\ sound\ in\ soft\ tissue}{ultrasound\ beam\ frequency} \qquad 6$$

Deducting from the equation it can be seen that the wavelength of the ultrasound beam is directly proportional to the speed of sound in soft tissue but inversely proportional to the frequency of the ultrasound beam. In this book, since the lower limb arteries to be examined were superficial structures, it, justified why the principal investigator chose the highest frequency linear probe of 7.5 - 10 MHz which was available for the ultrasound machine utilised in this book.

To ensure consistency the ultrasound parameters measurements were taken by the same rater (principal investigator) holding more than 5 years of experience in vascular ultrasound scanning. The principal investigator scanned, froze and measured the ultrasound parameters which included peak systolic velocity and pulsatility index from the still image of the spectral Doppler waveforms and the B-mode parameter which included vessel diameter inner to inner was measured from the still image of the longitudinal section of the popliteal arteries, anterior tibial arteries and posterior tibial arteries (Delis et al., 2000; Leoniuk et al., 2014). These measurements were performed three times for each participant and the mean value was recorded. The fact that the principal investigator held more than 5 years' experience in vascular imaging minimised performance bias during the undertaking of measurements and also the fact that a mean of three measurements was recorded also enabled minimisation of measurement error.

The principal investigator placed the ultrasound gel and then the linear probe over each artery for transverse scanning and then rotated 90^0 for the longitudinal scanning to enable the undertaking of Doppler and B mode measurements (Hwang, 2017; Eiberg et al., 2010).

The principal investigator sampled the blood flow for the arterial segments which include the popliteal arteries, anterior tibial arteries and posterior tibial arteries and dorsalis pedis arteries with B mode imaging, colour and then Doppler in the longitudinal section. The longitudinal section enabled the principal investigator to manipulate the ultrasound beam from the probe to be parallel to the blood flowing in the arteries thus enabling manoeuvring for a Doppler angle of less or equal to 60° which gives maximum Doppler shifts interpreted as the blood velocity on the Doppler spectral display (Hamments, 2014; Hwang, 2017). The principal investigator avoided sampling in the transverse section since it makes the ultrasound beam to be at 90° angle which gives zero Doppler shifts as the ultrasound beam will be traversing the arterial blood flow at right angles (Hamments, 2014; Hwang 2017). The principal investigator utilised the Doppler equation which identifies all factors affecting the magnitude of the Doppler shift as follows in equation 7;

$$FD = \frac{2ftv(\cos\theta)nx}{c} \qquad 7$$

From equation I,) FD refers to Doppler shift frequency (positive in arteries and negative in veins),

ii) 2 is a constant and can be ignored,

iii) Transmitted frequency *(FT)* is directly proportional to Doppler shift frequency *(FD)*.

iv) velocity of blood *(v)* is directly proportional Doppler shift frequency *(FD)* and *(C)* speed of sound which is 1.540 m/s and a constant (Hamments, 2014; Hwang 2017).

Deducting the Doppler equation above the principal investigator had to make sure that Doppler angle *(θ)* was less or equal to 60 to enable a cosine value that was high and which was directly proportional to high Doppler shifts which were also directly proportional to high blood velocity.

The principal investigator made the colour box as small as possible and placed the sample volume cursor within an arterial lumen to enable recording of more accurate and maximum Doppler shift frequencies. (Harrington, 2012; Chavhan et al., 2008). The Doppler spectrum then displayed the blood flow velocities in the y-axis in cm/s against time in seconds in the x-axis. See figure 8 for more detail on the correct placement of the sample volume cursor.

The pulsed spectral Doppler parameters including pulsatility index and resistive index were calculated automatically after the principal investigator measured the peak systolic velocity and end-diastolic velocity on the displayed spectral Doppler waveform in each arterial segment for each participant. See figure 5 for more detail of the measurement of Doppler parameters.

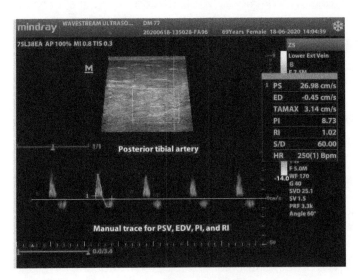

Figure 5 Measurement of Doppler ultrasound parameters within the posterior tibial artery performed by the principal investigator (Current book).

The principal investigator performed the measurements three times for each of the ultrasound parameters and recorded them under an anonymous code representing each participant. The scanning site for the right popliteal arteries was in the popliteal fossa region and the approach used to access it is shown in figure 6 and the arterial anatomy displayed in this position is shown in a Computed Tomography (CT) image in figure 8. In figure 6, the principal investigator positioned the patient supine and extended their right leg laterally and slightly abducted their knee joint medially.

The principal investigator placed the linear probe and sonar transmission gel over the popliteal region of the ankle and the Doppler scanning angle was maintained at $\leq 60°$ (Hwang, 2017; Eiberg et al., 2010). The principal investigator placed the probe over this region transversely to view the popliteal artery and vein lying side by side as confirmed by colour Doppler and, then rotated the probe 90° in-order to view the longitudinal section of the popliteal artery. The principal investigator gathered pulsed spectral Doppler and B-mode measurements for blood flow in the longitudinal section of the popliteal artery (Hwang, 2017; Eiberg et al., 2010; Leoniuk et al., 2014; Moneta et al., 1992).

The principal investigator undertook the scanning for the right anterior tibial arteries at its palpable pulse at the neck of the ankle slightly in front of the lateral malleolus (Hwang, 2017; Eiberg et al., 2010; Leoniuk et al., 2014). See figure 7 for more detail. The right dorsalis pedis arteries were accessed in the groove between the first and second phalanges while the right posterior tibial artery was accessed behind the medial malleolus (Hwang, 2017; Eiberg et al., 2010; Leoniuk et al., 2014) by the principal investigator and the ultrasound parameters were measured in these regions accordingly.

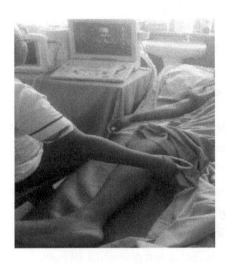

Figure 6 *Principal investigator demonstrating positioning technique for accessing the popliteal artery during ultrasound scanning (Current book.*

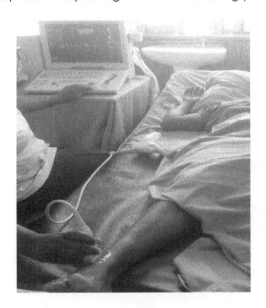

Figure 7 *Principal investigator demonstrating the scanning technique for accessing the right anterior tibial artery during ultrasound scanning. (Current book).*

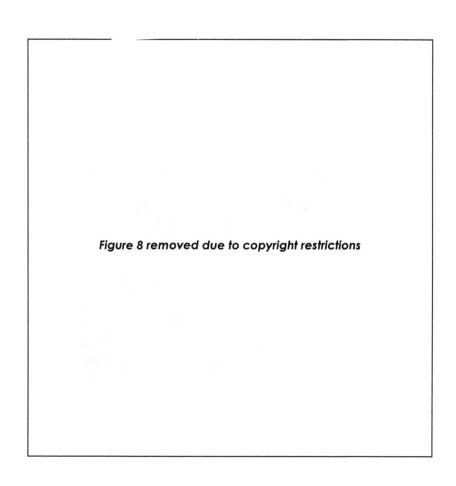

Figure 8 removed due to copyright restrictions

Figure 8 Computed Tomography Angiography image showing the arterial anatomy displayed with the patient supine and the leg extended, mildly abducted in the lateral position and slightly flexed (Hwang, 2017).

The principal investigator-assessed vessel diameter was performed in the greyscale image in the longitudinal section of the artery and obtained its measurements by placing the callipers on the inner to inner walls of the artery. In figure 12 vessel diameter inner to inner is labelled as VDI with a measurement of 0.54 cm in diameter. The principal investigator repeated this measurement process thrice for each vessel segment and recorded the mean value of the three measurements (Delis et al., 2000; Leoniuk et al., 2014).

The principal investigator did not include the vessel diameter outer to outer in this book, because prior evidence has shown vessel diameter inner to inner as more reproducible than vessel diameter outer to the outer (Hartshorne et al., 2011; Borgbderg et al., 2018). See figure 9 for more detail.

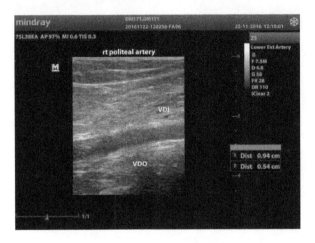

Figure 9 Measurements for vessel diameter inner to inner of the longitudinal section of a B-mode image of a popliteal artery segment, and vessel diameter outer to outer measurement also displayed (Current book).

3.9 Minimisation of measurement error during book data collection procedures

Quality control tests such as assessment of lateral resolution and axial resolution were carried out on the ultrasound machine by the PhD advisor to establish the machine's consistency in measurements during B-mode imaging to reduce the magnitude of error imaging measurements. This means that the magnitude of error in this investigation was solely from the measurement process itself and not from a faulty ultrasound scanner. A within sessions and between sessions repeatable study design was utilised leading to a mean value of three measurements of a parameter being recorded for each participant and this reduced the magnitude of measurement error.

3.10 Internal and external validity

The rigour in the design of each investigation of this book relied on participants' adherence to the rigorous diet restrictions outside the clinical set up before undergoing the measurements for blood flow, Ankle Brachial Index and blood pressure within clinical settings. However, measures which were put in place by the principal investigator for checking adherence to prior preparation diet made the three investigations to have high internal validity, and findings could be generalised to the Black /African diabetic population of Zimbabwe with early-stage PAD. However, external validity was limited because the strict inclusion and exclusion criteria put in place by the principal investigator did not allow recruitment of a diverse sample of participants belonging to other ethnic groups which generally represents the population of Zimbabwe.

Chapter 4 - First Investigation

Abstract

Repeatability of ultrasound parameters in measuring blood flow in the lower limb arteries of asymptomatic diabetic patients with early-stage PAD.

Keywords: *Doppler ultrasound imaging, Intraclass correlation coefficient, measurement error, B-mode vascular imaging*

Objectives: i) To determine the repeatability of ultrasound parameters in measuring lower limb blood flow in diabetic patients with early-stage PAD.

ii) To determine whether any differences in, dependent variables between sessions are significant or meaningful.

Methods: Ultrasound parameters consisting of peak systolic velocity (PSV), pulsatility index (PI), resistive index (RI) and vessel diameter inner to inner (VDI) were assessed for repeatability in measuring blood flow in the popliteal arteries (PA), anterior tibial arteries (ATA) and posterior tibial arteries (PTA) of 10 asymptomatic Black-African diabetic patients [3 *males, 7 females; mean age - 49.5 (13.8) years; mean* HbA_{1c} - *5.9 (0.7)%; mean - ABI 1.1 (0.1) and median BMI - 29.5 (24-33.7)*] with early-stage PAD. Both within sessions and between sessions reliability intraclass correlation coefficients (ICC), percentage coefficient of variation (%CV), standard error of measurement (SEM) and smallest detectable difference (SDD) were calculated for each parameter. Additionally, the paired *t*-test was performed to establish if any differences in, dependent variables between sessions were significant.

Results: All ultrasound parameters showed very good *(ICC ≥0.8; 0.6 – 0.9, 95% CI)* to excellent *(ICC ≤1.0; 1.0 – 1.0, 95% CI)* reliability and acceptably low variability *(≤5.6%CV)* both within and between sessions. Additionally, there were no significant or meaningful differences *(p ≥ 0.06; t ≥ -2.1)* between sessions for all the variables except VDI-PTA *(p = 0.03; t = -2.5)* and ATA *(p = 0.02; t = -2.9)*. The SEM was acceptably low *(SEM ≤1.1)* with low SDD (SDD <10%) for all parameters other than VDI-PTA (SDD = 13.6%).

Conclusions: Ultrasound parameters were repeatable in measuring blood flow in the lower limb arteries of diabetic patients with early-stage PAD and the associated measurement error was acceptably low, except VDI.

Correspondence to: Josephine S Tityiwe, National University of Science and Technology, Radiography Department, Corner Cecil/Gwanda Road, P. O. Box AC 939 Ascot, Bulawayo, Zimbabwe. Email: josephine.tityiwe@nust.ac.zw/ J.S.Tityiwe@edu.salford.ac.uk

4.1 Introduction

Prior evidence classified asymptomatic PAD as stage 1 by Fontaine et al., (1954) which refers to incomplete occlusion of arteries, while Rutherford et al., (1997) classified asymptomatic PAD as grade zero with additional objective data of being confirmed by a normal reactive hyperaemic test or treadmill test (Hardman et al., 2014). However, the classification for asymptomatic PAD by Fontaine et al., (1954) had a weakness of lacking objective data to rigorously rule out the probability of symptomatic PAD (Hardman et al., 2014). Prior evidence (Hirsch et al., 2005; Rooke et al., 2011; Gerhard-Herman et al., 2016), has recommended the utilisation of Ankle Brachial Index to quantify PAD and an Ankle Brachial Index value of greater or equal to 0.9 concluded to indicate symptomatic PAD. However, a numerical value of the Ankle Brachial Index is not able to provide the clinicians with the objective information on the clinical severity of the disease. This investigation aimed to contribute to the filling of this gap in the literature by determining the repeatability of duplex ultrasound parameters in measuring blood flow in the lower limbs of diabetic patients with early-stage PAD. The findings of this investigation could provide evidence for the drafting of management guidelines for diabetic patients with duplex ultrasound parameters whilst still in the secondary care of the Zimbabwean health delivery system.

In this investigation, the principal investigator combined ultrasound parameters including peak systolic velocity, pulsatility index, resistive index and vessel diameter inner to inner into a diagnostic protocol and tested them for repeatability in measuring blood flow in the lower limbs of asymptomatic diabetic patients with early-stage PAD. Although there is evidence showing that these ultrasound parameters have been widely used in the assessments of lower limb arteries blood flow for late-stage PAD (Eiberg et al., 2010; Andersen, 2010; Chen et al., 2015) this is the first time that these parameters have been combined this way. No prior studies which utilised ultrasound parameters to assess blood flow in asymptomatic diabetic patients with early-stage PAD were established during the writing up of this book. This investigation, therefore, aimed to provide evidence justifying the utilisation of duplex ultrasound parameters to assess blood flow in Black/African asymptomatic diabetic patients with early-stage PAD, which was objectively confirmed through a normal reactive hyperaemic test (Rutherford et al., 1997; Hardman et al., 2014).

4.2 Aims

i) To determine the within and between sessions reliability and measurement error of the ultrasound parameters in measuring blood flow in the lower limbs of diabetic patients with early-stage PAD.

ii) To determine if there were any significant or meaningful changes in, dependent variables (ultrasound blood parameters) between sessions.

4.2.1 Research Questions

i) Can the ultrasound parameters repeatably measure blood flow in the lower limb arteries of diabetic patients with early-stage PAD?

ii) Are the differences in, dependent variables between sessions significant or meaningful?

4.3 Methodology

4.3.1 Design

The design for this investigation is outlined in section 3.3 of this book while in this investigation, the ultrasound parameters measurements were made by the same instrument (same sonar machine), same rater (principal investigator) under identical conditions in the two sessions. The principal investigator performed these measurements within a short lapse period of only 1 week (Scanlon, 2012), to avoid any probable changes in the participants' health state which could have altered the responses they elicited during first session measurements (Kimberlin, 2008; Shuttleworth, 2009). In this case, the lapse period of one week between the measurements sessions would not have allowed a significant accumulation of PAD which could alter basal blood flow in the participants' lower limb arteries. This measure enabled minimisation of measurement error between sessions.

4.3.2 Participants

The principal investigator, assessed both within and between sessions reliability and measurement error to determine if ultrasound parameters could repeatably measure blood flow in thirty arterial segments of the right lower limbs of 10 Black-African diabetic patients [3 males, 7 females; mean age - 49.5 (13.8) years; mean HbA_{1c} - 5.86 (0.7) %; mean - ABI 1.1 (0.1) and median BMI - 29.5 (24-33.7)] with early-stage PAD. All the participants in this investigation provided written informed consent for participation and the Medical Research Council of Zimbabwe and Salford ethics board approved the study.

The principal investigator's justification for the inclusion and exclusion criteria for the participants is outlined in section 3.4 in the methods section for this book, while the prior patient preparation requirements are outlined in section 3.6 in chapter 3 the methods section.

The principal investigator utilised the classification for early-stage PAD by Rutherford et al., (1997), "the asymptomatic grade zero" (Hardman et al., 2014), in the randomised recruitment of the 10 diabetic participants from Mpilo central hospital's diabetic clinic in the city of Bulawayo, Zimbabwe. Participants who did not illicit a decrease or who elicited a small decrease in ankle blood pressure at rest following reactive hyperaemia tests by the diabetic clinic-based physician were included. All the diabetic patients who did not qualify to be categorised as having early-stage PAD according to the inclusion criteria were no longer eligible for this investigation but were left to continue with their care with the physician in the diabetic clinic. Therefore, the principal investigator highlighted this important instruction in the information sheets given to the patients before consenting to participate in this investigation to ensure that non-qualifying patients would not be confused and discontinue their routine treatments. This process enabled minimisation of bias due to misclassification of exposure and outcomes because the rigorous screening of diabetic patients with the reactive hyperaemic test enabled the selection of participants with early-stage PAD (the exposure factor) while those in later stages of PAD were excluded.

4.4 Data collection procedures

4.4.1 Reactive Hyperaemic testing and sampling

The research assistants utilised the inclusion and exclusion criteria in section 3.4 of chapter 3 to randomly recruit volunteering participants who were to undergo reactive hyperaemic testing in the physician's room at the diabetic clinic.

The research assistants assigned the recruited volunteering participants with anonymous identification codes and allowed them 10 minutes rest in the diabetic clinic to enable them to get a stable heart rate before undergoing hyperaemic testing in the physician's room. The research assistants then escorted each of the volunteering participants into the physician's room where the physician performed reactive hyperaemic testing on the right leg of each of them in the presence of the principal investigator. Despite its documented weakness of causing mild discomfort in diabetic patients, the principal investigator chose the reactive hyperaemic test for this investigation since, its equipment was affordable within the budget of this book compared to the treadmill test equipment (Higashi et al., 2001; Philpott and Anderson, 2007).

The research assistants booked the ten participants who were categorised as having early-stage PAD on day 5 to undergo blood tests in the laboratory and ultrasound measurements at a private ultrasound imaging centre in the city of Bulawayo. The research assistants assigned the recruited participants with anonymous identification codes and put them on detailed prior preparation instructions to address their diet for three days and absconding their medication first thing in the morning before undertaking of blood tests and ultrasound measurements. See section 3.6 in chapter 3 for more detail.

4.4.2 Blood testing for renal function and glycaemic control

Blood tests were done first at 8 0'clock in the morning of day 5 in the laboratory and ultrasound measurements were done soon after blood tests downstairs in the same building by the principal investigator. The participants' blood was tested for glycated haemoglobin levels to establish glycaemic control in the recruited participants. Again, the blood was tested for Urea and Creatinine levels which were utilised to calculate the Estimated Glomerular Filtration Rate to establish whether the recruited participants indeed had minimal renal damage as supposedly expected in early-stage PAD. The principal investigator used these blood tests as medical history demographic markers confirming that the prior reactive hyperaemic test had been effectively utilised to recruit diabetic patients with early-stage PAD as reflected by effective glycaemic control and minimal renal damage.

See appendices E1 to E4 for evidence of the blood test results undertaken on the diabetic patients in the laboratory. The blood test results were availed by the laboratory the following day (Day 6) and the research assistants stratified the recruited 10 anonymised coded participants with their blood tests results while this was blinded to the principal investigator to minimise recall bias.

4.4.3 Doppler ultrasound parameters and Ankle Brachial Index measurements

The quality control tests undertaken for the ultrasound scanner which included internal grid assessment for testing lateral and axial resolution for the 7.5-10.0 MHz probe are outlined in section 3.8 while the quality control tests for the Blood pressure machine which included calibration are outlined in section 3.7.

All the recruited 10 volunteers were escorted from the laboratory by the research assistants to the ultrasound room downstairs on day 5. In the ultrasound room, the participants were assessed in quiet, calm conditions at standard room temperature of about 23 - 25°C by a thermometer.

Weight and height of the participants were measured by the research assistants who then stratified it with the participants' anonymised codes on Microsoft Excel sheets. The principal investigator later calculated the body mass index for the recorded weight and height of each patient and stratified it alongside the anonymised codes. See section 3.7 of chapter 3 for more detail on body mass index calculations which were undertaken.

The principal investigator performed Ankle Brachial Index as outlined in section 3.7 of chapter 3 on the 10 participants and the research assistants recorded and collated the Ankle Brachial Index results for each patient with the anonymised codes in Microsoft Excel sheets.

Again, the principal investigator performed B-mode imaging and measured vessel diameter inner to inner followed by duplex ultrasound parameters measurements for peak systolic velocity and end-diastolic velocity which enabled automatic calculation of resistive index and pulsatility index by the ultrasound machine. See section 3.8 for more detail on the scanning technique undertaken by the principal investigator.

The research assistants gave the participants some refreshments before dismissing them to go home with bookings and prior preparation instructions (Section 3.6) to be followed before retesting by the principal investigator after 1 week.

Personalised contact was maintained by research assistants with patients through prompt text messages and telephone calls to remind patients of the prior dietary preparations before their appointment for session 2 duplex ultrasound measurements. This measure enabled the minimisation of transfer bias (Paccunni and Wilkins, 2010) between the two sessions.

The quality control tests for the ultrasound scanner (section 3.8) which were done before the undertaking of session 1 were repeated before the undertaking of session 2.

During the second session, the demographic data and Ankle Brachial Index findings of the diabetic patients were simply imported from the first session, while the blood tests were not repeated since they were simply demographic markers confirming early-stage PAD which had already been confirmed through prior reactive hyperaemic testing.

The principal investigator repeated the duplex ultrasound measurements which were done in session 1 after one week (Scanlon, 2012) as outlined in section 3.8 of this book to avoid incurring any probable changes in the patients' health state which could alter the responses which they had initially elicited during session 1 measurements (Kimberlin, 2008), such as progression of PAD if re-testing were to be done after a long time frame.

The principal investigator was blinded to the results of the first session measurements while performing the second session measurements and the research assistants documented the archived measurements for the first and second sessions. Thus, each time the principal investigator scanned and stored the data in the archives of the sonar machine the research assistants later collected the data and inputted it into simple excel tables tallying the scan findings of each patient with their session 1 findings. This process minimised recall bias which could have occurred if the principal investigator collated the data findings (Paccunni and Wilkins, 2010).

In this investigation, the shorter time frame between sessions 1 and 2 minimised the likeliness of patients moving away from the research site in pursuit of other personal reasons, See section 4.3.1 for more detail on the justification for this shorter time frame.

4.4.4 Decision making during data collection

During the collection of data for this investigation, the principal investigator discovered that the longitudinal section of the dorsalis pedis arteries borders was not so clear or definite to allow repeatable and consistent measurements of vessel diameter inner to inner when compared to the posterior tibial artery, anterior tibial artery and popliteal artery vessels. See figures 10 and 11 for the detailed illustration. Therefore, the principal investigator decided to exclude the assessment of the dorsalis pedis artery preliminarily since all the ultrasound parameters making up the diagnostic protocol in this investigation were to be assessed for repeatability in measuring blood flow in the lower limb arteries. The principal investigator then focussed on assessing the popliteal arteries, anterior tibial arteries and posterior tibial arteries.

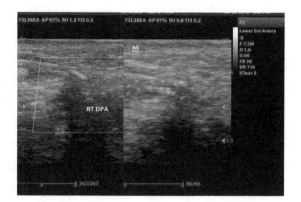

Figure 10 *longitudinal section of the right dorsalis pedis and the inner to inner borders of the artery not so clear in the B - mode image to the right (Current book).*

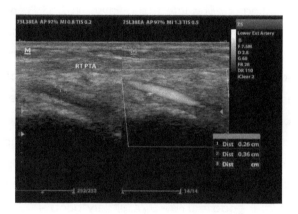

Figure 11 *longitudinal section of the posterior tibial artery and the inner to inner borders of the artery clearly shown allowing the measurements to be consistent in the B-mode image to the left (Current book).*

4.5 Statistical analyses

The principal investigator utilised the Shapiro-Wilks test (Shapiro and Wilks, 1965) to check for normality of the demographic data which included the diabetic patients' characteristics before further analysis of the data from the ultrasound parameters measurements. The justification for utilising the Shapiro-Wilks test by the principal investigator was because statistical methods are more precise in detecting normality than graphical methods since actual probabilities that the sample was drawn from a normal population are calculated besides also being more sensitive in detecting non-normality in smaller samples of n < 100 (Zaiontz, 2013-2017). See table 2 for information on the demographic data for the first investigation.

The principal investigator conducted all analyses in SPSS (Version 16.0; SPSS, Inc., IL, USA) and then computed firstly the Intraclass correlation coefficient (ICC) values from within sessions single measurements for each ultrasound parameter which they performed thrice to enable the calculation of ICC for within-session reliability with the associated 95% confidence interval and secondly, the principal investigator calculated the mean of the three trials of day one and the mean of the three trials on day two and computed them to enable the calculation of ICC for between-sessions reliability with its associated 95% confidence interval. The principal investigator then classified the ICC as follows; i) good = 0.60 - 0.74; ii) very good = 0.75 - 0.89 and iii) excellent ≥90, based on the lower bound confidence interval (Koo and Li, 2016). An *a priori* alpha level was set at $p \leq 0.05$ (Paccunni and Wilkins, 2010; Karras, 1997). The principal investigator did this in a bid to try and answer the first research question for this investigation which sought to establish if the ultrasound parameters could repeatably measure blood flow in the diabetic lower limb arteries with early-stage PAD. The ICC parameter used by the principal investigator as a within and between sessions reliability correlation to quantify repeatability of the ultrasound parameters in this investigation had a weakness of showing a correlation only within sessions not between sessions (days), again if a measure increased or decreased by the same magnitude in all subjects then the ICC value may indicate that the measure is reliable, even though there could be a significant and meaningful change between sessions (days) (Paccunni and Wilkins, 2010; Karras, 1997). Therefore, the principal investigator utilised the paired *t*-test (XU et al., 2017; Paccunni and Wilkins, 2010) to determine whether there was statistical evidence suggesting that the mean difference between the paired measurements of the two sessions was significantly different from zero or not thus demonstrating the robustness of the measuring instrument. The hypothesis utilised here by the principal investigator was that there was no significant difference between the paired measurements of the two sessions (days). Therefore, a statistically significant difference in the ultrasound parameters measurements between sessions would thus mean that the measurements were not stable over the two sessions. The principal investigator did this in a bid to try and answer the second research question of this investigation which sought to determine if there were any significant differences in dependent variables (ultrasound blood flow parameters) between sessions.

The principal investigator did not utilise Cohen's *d* weighting since they measured the same sample of diabetic patients under the same conditions over the two sessions, thus the samples were dependent.

The principal investigator quantified the variability in this investigation which could have been due to physiological differences between sessions/ days as a percentage coefficient of variation (%CV) to establish the variability of the ultrasound parameters amongst individuals, the mean and standard deviations (SDs) across the three trials for each individual were calculated then percentage coefficient of variation (%CV) for each individual was calculated and expressed as an average for the 10 participants. However, to establish the variability of the ultrasound parameters measurements between the two visiting sessions, the principal investigator calculated the mean (SDs) across the average for session one and two and then calculated the %CV for session one and session two. Then the principal investigator put good reliability in this investigation at an upper limit of <10%CV, thus in comparison with previously established %CV values reporting good reliability (Thomas et al., 2015; Cormack et al., 2008; Sheppard et al., 2011).

The principal investigator calculated the standard error of measurement (SEM) between sessions using the following formula in equation 8;

$$SEM = SD\ (first\ observed) \times \sqrt{1} - ICC\ (first\ observed), \qquad 8$$

Accordingly, the principal investigator calculated the smallest detectable difference (SDD) between sessions to determine the associated magnitude of measurement error using the following formula in equation 9;

$$SDD = Z\ \text{score}\ (95\%\ CI) \times SEM \times \sqrt{2}\ \text{ thus } SDD = 1.96 \times SEM \times \sqrt{2} \qquad 9$$

(Lee et al., 2013; Thomas et al., 2015; Sheppard et al., 2011).

4.6 Results

4.6.1 Demographic findings

In a cohort of 10 Black-African participants with early-stage PAD, 3 (30%) were males and 7 (70%) were females (Table 2). The demographic results showed that glycated haemoglobin levels, age and the Ankle Brachial Index were normally distributed, thus the principal investigator analysed them as means (SD)s, while the Body Mass Index and Estimated Glomerular Filtration rate were not normally distributed thus, these the principal investigator analysed as median interquartile ranges (IQR)s (Table 2).

Table 2 Descriptive statistics for demographic findings for a cohort of diabetic patients with early-stage PAD, (n = 10).

Variable	Normality test p-value	Mean (SD)	Median (IQR)
EGFR	0.0		105.0 (93.0 -116.0) ml/min/1.73 m^2
HbA$_{1c}$	0.6	6.0 (0.7)%	
BMI	0.0		30.0 (24.0 – 34.0)
Age	0.8	50.0 (14.0) years	
ABI	0.9	1.1 (0.1)	

4.6.2 The Popliteal artery (PA) findings

Peak systolic velocity, pulsatility index, resistive index and vessel diameter inner to inner showed very good to excellent reliability both within and between sessions with acceptably low variability both within and between sessions and an acceptably low Smallest Detectable Difference (SDD%) (Table 3a) Additionally, the difference between sessions for measurements for all the ultrasound parameters was equal to zero and not significant (Table 3b).

Table 3a Descriptive and reliability statistics of ultrasound parameters in the popliteal artery (PA) (n= 10).

Variable	Mean (SD)		ICC (95% CI)		% CV		Measurement error	
	Session 1	Session 2	Within session	Between sessions	Within sessions	Between sessions	SEM	SDD (SDD %)
PSV - PA	59.3 (9.0) cm/s	60.0 (8.4) cm/s	1.0 (1.0 – 1.0)	1.0 (1.0 – 1.0)	0.1%	0.3%	0.0	0.0 (0.0%)
PI-PA	6.0 (1.4)	6.0 (1.3)	0.9 (0.8 - 1.0)	1.0 (1.0 - 1.0)	0.1%	0.9%	0.1	0.4 (6.6%)
RI-PA	1.0 (0.0)	1.0 (0.0)	0.9 (0.7 - 1.0)	1.0 (1.0 - 1.0)	0.3%	0.5%	0.0	0.0 (3.0%)
VDI-PA	0.5 (0.1) cm	0.5 (0.1) cm	1.0 (1.0 - 1.0)	1.0 (1.0 - 1.0)	0.1%	0.5%	0.0	0.0 (0.0%)

SD = standard deviation; ICC = intraclass correlation coefficient; %CV = percentage coefficient of variation; SDD = smallest detectable difference; SEM = standard error of measurement; n = sample size. PSV = peak systolic velocity; PI = pulsatility index; RI = resistive index; VDI = vessel diameter inner to inner; PA = popliteal artery

Table 3b *Descriptive and between sessions comparisons of ultrasound parameters in the Popliteal Arteries (n = 10)*

Vessel parameter	Mean (SD) session 1	Mean(SD) session 2	Mean difference	t- value	Degrees of freedom	2 tailed p-value	95% CI day 1	95% CI day 2
PSV-PA	59.3 (8.0) cm/s	60.0 (9.0) cm/s	-0.3	-2.1	9	0.1	53.0; 66.0	53.3; 66.0
PI – PA	6 (2.0)	5.0 (1.3)	0.1	0.3	9	0.8	4.9; 7.0	5; 7.0
RI-PA	1.0 (0.0)	1.0 (0.0)	0.0	1.4	9	0.2	1.0; 1.0	1.0; 1.0
VDI – PA	0.5 (0.1) cm	0.5 (0.1) cm	0.0	1.5	9	0.2	0.4; 0.6	0.4; 0.6

SD= standard deviation; *t*-value = *t*- test statistic; CI = confidence interval; n = sample size; PSV = peak systolic velocity; PI = pulsatility index; RI = resistive index; VDI = vessel diameter inner to inner; PA = popliteal artery

4.6.3 The anterior tibial artery (ATA) Findings

Peak systolic velocity, pulsatility index, resistive index and vessel diameter inner to inner showed very good to excellent reliability both within and between sessions and acceptably low variability both within and between sessions and the associated Smallest Detectable Difference was acceptably low (Table 4a). Additionally, the difference between days of measurements for all the ultrasound parameters was equal to zero and not significant except vessel diameter inner to inner which showed a significant difference between sessions (Table 4b).

Table 4a Descriptive statistics and within and between sessions reliability of ultrasound parameters in the anterior tibial artery (ATA) (n = 10).

Variable	Mean (SD)		ICC (95%CI)		%CV		SEM	SDD (SDD %)
	Session 1	Session 2	Within session	Between sessions	Within sessions	Between sessions		
PSV - ATA	44.4 (9.2) cm/s	44.4 (9.0) cm/s	1.0 (1.0 - 1.0)	1.0 (1.0 - 1.0)	1.1%	0.1%	0.0	0.0 (0.0%)
PI - ATA	7.9 (2.1)	7.8 (1.8)	1.0 (1.0 - 1.0)	1.0 (1.0 - 1.0)	0.7%	0.6%	0.0	0.0 (0.0%)
RI - ATA	1.0 (0.1)	1.0 (0.1)	1.0 (0.9 - 1.0)	1.0 (1.0 - 1.0)	0.3%	0.9%	0.0	0.0 (3.0%)
VDI - ATA	0.2 (0.0) cm	0.2 (0.0) cm	0.8 (0.6 – 0.9)	1.0 (0.9 - 1.0)	5.6%	3.6%	0.00	0.0 (0.0%)

SD = standard deviation; ICC = intraclass correlation coefficient; %CV = percentage coefficient of variation; SDD = smallest detectable difference; SEM = standard error of measurement; PSV = peak systolic velocity, PI = pulsatility index; RI = resistive index; VDI = vessel diameter inner to inner

Table 4b *Descriptive statistics and between sessions comparisons of ultrasound parameters in the anterior tibial arteries (n = 10)*

Vessel parameter	Mean (SD) Session 1	Mean (SD) session 2	Mean difference	t-value	Degrees of freedom	2 tailed p-value	95% CI session 1	95% CI session 2
PSV - ATA	44.4 (9.6)	44.4 (9.3)	-0.0	-0.2	9	0.9	37.5; 51.2	37.7; 51.1
PI – ATA	7.9 (2.1)	7.8 (1.9)	0.1	0.5	9	0.6	6.4; 9.4	6.5; 9.2
RI - ATA	1.0 (0.1)	1.0 (0.1)	0.0	1.3	9	0.2	0.9; 1.1	0.9; 1.1
VDI - ATA	0.2 (0.0)	0.2 (0.0)	-0.0	**-2.9**	9	**0.0**	0.2; 0.2	0.2; 0.2

SD= standard deviation; t-value = t- test statistic; CI = confidence interval; n = sample size; PSV = peak systolic velocity, PI = pulsatility index; RI = resistive index; VDI = vessel diameter inner to inner.

4.6.4 The posterior tibial artery (PTA) findings

Peak systolic velocity, pulsatility index, resistive index and vessel diameter inner to inner showed very good to excellent reliability and acceptably low variability both within and between sessions and the associated Smallest Detectable Difference was acceptably low except for vessel diameter inner to inner where Smallest Detectable Difference was unacceptably high (table 5a). Additionally, the difference between days of measurements for all the ultrasound parameters was equal to zero and not significant except for vessel diameter inner to inner which showed a significant difference between sessions (Table 5b).

Table 5a *Descriptive statistics and within and between sessions reliability of ultrasound parameters in the posterior tibial artery (PTA) (n = 10).*

Variable	Mean (SD)		ICC (95% CI)		%CV		SEM	SDD (SDD %)
	Session 1	Session 2	Within session	Between sessions	Within sessions	Between sessions		
PSV-PTA	39.8 (11) cm/s	39.7 (11) cm/s	0.9 (0.8 - 1.0)	1.0 (1.0 - 1.0)	1.7%	0.1%	1.1	3.0 (7.6%)
PI - PTA	5.8 (1.4)	5.8 (1.3)	1.0 (0.9 - 1.0)	1.0 (1.0 - 1.0)	3.9%	0.3%	0.1	0.4 (6.6%)
RI - PTA	1.1 (0.2)	1.1 (0.1)	0.9 (0.8 - 1.0)	1.0 (1.0 - 1.0)	3.6%	0.6%	0.0	0.1 (5.9%)
VDI - PTA	0.2 (0.1) cm	0.2 (0.0) cm	1.0 (0.9 - 1.0)	1.0 (1.0 - 1.0)	4.8%	2.3%	0.0	**0.0 (13.6%)**

SD = standard deviation; ICC = intraclass correlation coefficient; %CV = percentage coefficient of variation; SDD = smallest detectable difference; SEM = standard error of measurement; PSV = peak systolic velocity, PI = pulsatility index; RI = resistive index; VDI = vessel diameter inner to inner.

Table 5b *Descriptive statistics and between sessions comparisons of ultrasound parameters in the posterior tibial arteries (n = 10)*

Vessel parameter	Mean (SD) Session 1	Mean (SD) Session 2	Mean difference	t-value	Degrees of freedom	2 tailed p-value	95% CI session 1	95% CI session 2
PSV-PTA	39.8 (11.3) cm/s	39.7 (11.1) cm/s	-0.1	0.3	9	0.8	31.7; 47.9	31.8; 47.6
PI-PTA	5.9 (1.4)	5.8 (1.4)	0.0	0.3	9	0.8	4.9; 6.8	4.8; 6.8
RI-PTA	1.1 (0.2)	1.1 (0.1)	0.0	0.5	9	0.6	1.0; 1.2	1.0; 1.1
VDI-PTA	0.2 (0.1)	0.2 (0.1)	-0.0	**-2.5**	9	**0.0**	0.2; 0.3	0.2; 0.3

SD = standard deviation; *t* - value = *t* - test statistic; CI = confidence interval; n = sample size; PSV = peak systolic velocity, PI = pulsatility index; RI = resistive index; VDI = vessel diameter inner to inner.

4.7 Discussion

In this investigation, the ultrasound parameters consisting of peak systolic velocity, pulsatility index, resistive index and vessel diameter inner to inner showed good repeatability in measuring blood flow in the lower limbs of diabetic patients with early-stage PAD which reflected as good (ICC ≥0.8; 0.6 – 0.9, 95% CI) to excellent (ICC ≤1.0; 1.0 – 1.0, 95% CI) reliability, low variability (≤5.6% CV), small measurement error (SEM ≤1.09) and small magnitude of measurement error (SDD <10%) with the exclusion of vessel diameter inner to inner for the posterior tibial artery (SDD% = 13.6%). Additionally, the difference between the two sessions of measurements for all the ultrasound parameters was not significant, except for vessel diameter inner to inner for the posterior tibial arteries which showed a higher magnitude of measurement error (SDD% = 13.6%) and a significant difference between sessions (p = 0.0; t = -2.5). Similarly, the anterior tibial arteries which showed a significant difference between sessions (p = 0.0; t = -2.9).

Deducting from the SEM equation; $SEM = SD\ (first\ observed) \times \sqrt{1} - ICC$ (first observed), it can be seen that measurements show an SEM closer to zero, thus SDD% ≤10% when reliability is 1.0 thus there will be no errors of measurement with a perfectly reliable test while a set of errors all equal to zero have no variability (Harvill, 2019). Similarly, these findings were obtained by Thomas et al., (2015); Sheppard et al., (2011) in their studies with different populations as well. The findings of this investigation reflected a low SEM of ≤1.1 (SDD ≤10%) in all the measurements of the ultrasound parameters except for vessel diameter inner to inner for the posterior tibial arteries which showed an unacceptably high SDD% (13.6%).

No prior evidence was found justifying the utilisation of ultrasound parameters to quantify or screen for early-stage PAD in asymptomatic diabetic patients or non-diabetic participants during the writing up of this book. One study by

Leoniuk et al., (2014), utilised Doppler and B-mode ultrasound parameters to compare blood flow in the posterior tibial arteries and dorsalis pedis arteries of diabetic Polish participants with early-stage PAD with a non-diabetic control group and they established no significant difference in the measurements for the Doppler ultrasound between the two groups ($p > 0.05$). In their study, Leoniuk et al., (2014) did not show evidence which tested the robustness of their ultrasound tool before utilising it in measuring lower limb blood flow in a larger sample of their study to minimise on measurement error. The prior assessment of measurement error of a measurement tool is important to show the evidence that the tool can be able to accurately measure clinically significant changes which can show effects of an intervention on patients (Lee et al., 2013). Again, a small magnitude of the measurement error in a tool increases the confidence of using this tool to screen for pathology in larger sample populations (Lee et al., 2013). The generalisability of the findings of the study by Leoniuk et al., (2014) was not clear based on the fact that there was no clear description of the population studied in Poland i.e. whether the population was homogeneous or heterogeneous.

In this investigation, the ultrasound parameters including peak systolic velocity, resistive index, and pulsatility index showed a small SEM and a small SDD% except for vessel diameter inner to inner for the anterior tibial arteries and the posterior tibial arteries. These findings reflected the evidence that peak systolic velocity, resistive index and pulsatility index can detect a clinically significant change in the lower limb blood flow resulting from early-stage PAD with the exclusion of vessel diameter inner to inner due to more measurement errors.

Again, bias due to the misclassification of exposure and outcomes was not minimised in the methodology of the study by Leoniuk et al., (2014) for no controls were put in place to limit the effects of nitrate enriched diets, blood pressure reducing medications or alcohol and this could have affected basal blood flow in the participants before the undertaking of Doppler ultrasound measurements and this could have contributed to error in their measurements.

The categorisation for early-stage by Leoniuk et al., (2014), utilised PAD grading undertaken by Fontaine et al., (1954) which classified early stage (asymptomatic) PAD in the category of incomplete blood vessel obstruction. However, the weakness of the PAD classification by Fontaine et al., (1954) is that it does not provide objective data which rules out the probability of symptomatic PAD. This was accordingly revealed in the findings of Leoniuk et al., (2014) which then showed 41 out of 148 arterial segments which had Doppler ultrasound waveforms with the biphasic flow and 4 out of 148 arterial segments which had Doppler waveforms with monophasic flow reflecting the presence of haemodynamically significant changes of symptomatic PAD amongst their participants.

In this investigation, the grading for PAD was done utilising the classification by Rutherford et al., (1997) which classified early-stage PAD as asymptomatic grade zero which is confirmed by objective data of a normal reactive hyperaemic test or treadmill test. All the diabetic patients in this investigation underwent reactive hyperaemic testing to strengthen the objectivity of grading for early-stage PAD and all the ultrasound Doppler waveforms of the participants' arterial segments showed normal triphasic flow reflecting evidence of non- haemodynamically significant changes in early-stage PAD.

4.8 Strengths and Limitations

The findings of this investigation had limited external validity because due to a limited budget, the principal investigator was not able to draw a wider heterogeneous sample size representing the Zimbabwean population such that these findings will only be generalised to Zimbabwean Black/African diabetic patients with early-stage PAD.

In this investigation, the principal investigator utilised Body Mass Index to establish the health status of the diabetic patients though it had a weakness of not being able to differentiate weight from fat or muscle. This was because the budget of the book was limited and could not afford better tools for assessing body fat e.g. from skinfold thickness measurements. Thus, in this book, the principal investigator utilised Body Mass Index as a screening tool for body fatness in the participants but not as a diagnostic tool.

The principal investigator utilised reactive hyperaemic testing was utilised for screening for early-stage PAD in the asymptomatic diabetic patients despite prior evidence of it causing mild discomfort in the participants, this was because of the limited budget of the book which could not afford a treadmill.

During the gathering of data, the principal investigator dropped the assessment of the dorsalis pedis arteries since the measurements for vessel diameter inner to inner were not consistently reproducible. Therefore, she decided to stop the further analysis of the dorsalis pedis artery in the second investigation.

The strength of this investigation was that it was carried out with some controls put in place by the principal investigator to minimise recall, performance and misclassification of exposure and outcomes bias as well as measurement error (Paccunni and Wilkins, 2010). Again, the other control put in place by the principal investigator was the objective screening for early-stage PAD using reactive hyperaemic testing to reduce measurement error by recruiting diabetic patients with a similar stage of PAD.

The other strength of this investigation was that the principal investigator determined the repeatability of the measurement method under controlled settings to establish its robustness before utilisation it with a bigger sample of participants in the second and third investigations of this book.

4.9 Conclusions and recommendations

Based on the findings of this investigation, the principal investigator concluded that ultrasound parameters which include peak systolic velocity, pulsatility index and resistive index were repeatable in measuring the effects of early-stage PAD on the lower limb blood flow of asymptomatic Zimbabwean

Black/African diabetic patients with no significant or meaningful differences between sessions except vessel diameter inner to inner.

In this investigation, the principal investigator, therefore, recommended that peak systolic velocity, pulsatility index and resistive index be utilised side by side with Ankle Brachial Index in screening and quantifying early-stage PAD in asymptomatic diabetic patients.

4.10 Implications

The principal investigator deducted the implications of this investigation as that the ultrasound parameters such which include peak systolic velocity, pulsatility index and resistive index form a robust diagnostic protocol for demonstrating the effects of early-stage PAD on lower limb blood flow of asymptomatic Black/African Zimbabwean diabetic patients.

4.11 Decision making for the second investigation

The principal investigator decided to import peak systolic velocity, pulsatility index and resistive index into the second investigation to compare blood flow in the lower limb arteries of non-diabetic participants and asymptomatic diabetic patients with early-stage PAD due to their robustness shown in this investigation. The principal investigator also decided to drop vessel diameter inner to inner from further assessments of blood flow between groups in the second investigation due to more errors in measurements and instability between sessions.

Chapter 5 – Second Investigation

Abstract

Comparison of key ultrasound variables between the diabetic lower limb arteries with early-stage Peripheral Artery Disease and non-diabetic controls.

Keywords: Atherosclerosis, peak systolic velocity, pulsatility index, resistive index.

Objectives: i) To compare lower limb blood flow in asymptomatic diabetic patients with early-stage peripheral artery disease (PAD) and non-diabetic controls using duplex ultrasound parameters.

ii) To determine if there were any significant or meaningful differences in, dependent variables (ultrasound parameters) between groups.

Methods: A comparative cohort study of lower limb blood flow in 35 Black-African diabetic patients *(25 females and 10 males)* with early-stage PAD and 36 -non-diabetic controls *(28 females and 8 males); median age 54 (IQR, 47 – 61) years; median HbA_{1c} 6.3 (IQR, 5.7 – 8.0)%; mean BMI 29.2 (± 6.7); mean ABI 1.1 (± 0.1)*. Robust ultrasound parameters from the first investigation which included peak systolic velocity (PSV), pulsatility index (PI) and resistive index (RI), were utilised to compare blood flow in the popliteal arteries (PA), anterior tibial arteries (ATA) and posterior tibial arteries (PTA) between groups while Ankle Brachial Index was measured and compared between groups as a parallel test.

Results: the ultrasound parameters consisting of PSV, RI and PI were significantly and meaningfully higher *(P <0.001; d ≥0.3)*, in diabetic patients compared to non-diabetic controls except for PI - PTA *(P = 0.7; d = 0.1)*. All the ultrasound parameters showed good *(ICC ≥0.7; 0.5 – 0.85, 95% CI)* to excellent *(ICC ≥1.0; 1.0 – 1.0, 95% CI)* within groups as well as acceptable variability *(<10% CV)* within groups other than pulsatility index of the anterior tibial artery within diabetic patients *(11.1%CV)*.

Conclusions: Ultrasound parameters including PSV and RI demonstrated a difference in lower limb blood flow between diabetic patients with early-stage PAD and non-diabetic controls. Thus, these parameters were able to highlight the effects of early-stage PAD on lower limb blood flow of diabetic patients. However, the effects of early-stage PAD on blood flow were not demonstrated in the PTA and ATA of diabetic patients by PI.

Correspondence to: Josephine S Tityiwe, National University of Science and Technology, Radiography Department, Corner Cecil/Gwanda Road, P. O. Box AC 939 Ascot, Bulawayo, Zimbabwe. Email: josephine.tityiwe@nust.ac.zw/ J.S.Tityiwe@edu.salford.ac.uk

5.1 Introduction

Prior studies on PAD have shown a high prevalence of asymptomatic PAD in the primary health care set up (Fowkes et al., 1991; Criqui et al., 1985), Therefore, enhanced early detection of PAD in patients at risk for PAD and cardiovascular diseases such as diabetics is essential to enable earlier initiation of treatment to delay the patients' from sliding into late-stage PAD symptoms such as critical limb ischaemia and gangrene.

Current guidelines (Rooke et al, 2011; Hirsh et al., 2005; Gerhard-Herman et al., 2016) have recommended Ankle Brachial Index for the screening and quantification of asymptomatic PAD and this is even though Ankle Brachial Index is not able to provide objective information on the clinical severity of the disease to the referring clinician. The aim of this investigation was therefore to establish the capability of duplex ultrasound parameters in detecting the effects of early-stage PAD on the blood flow of asymptomatic Black/ African Zimbabwean diabetic patients. The justification for the undertaking of this investigation being that no prior study was done showing evidence on the utilisation of duplex ultrasound this way. Thus, this investigation aimed to show whether duplex ultrasound modality can be utilised to augment the findings of Ankle Brachial Index in the screening and quantification of early-stage PAD which causes less than 50% stenosis in the lower limb arteries of Black/African asymptomatic diabetic patients.

Prior studies have shown that ultrasound parameters demonstrate high sensitivity (80 - 98%) and specificity (89 - 99%) in detecting late-stage PAD which causes $\geq$ 50% arterial lumen stenosis in diabetic patients (Collins et al., 2007; Type 2 Diabetes in adults: management (NG 28), NICE 2015; Di Minno et al., 2014; Carthy, 2013). However, during the writing up of this book, no evidence was found on the utilisation of duplex ultrasound to assess the effects of early-stage PAD on the lower limbs arterial blood flow of Black/ African diabetic patients in Zimbabwe and neither was there any documented evidence on the sensitivity or specificity of ultrasound parameters in detecting effects of early-stage PAD on blood flow. This investigation aimed to fill this literature gap by utilising duplex ultrasound parameters which include peak systolic velocity, pulsatility index and resistive index which came out as robust from the first investigation to compare blood flow in asymptomatic diabetic patients with early-stage PAD with non-diabetic controls in a bid to answer the first research question of this investigation. The second research question for this investigation was to establish if there could be a significant difference in blood flow between the groups which could be interpreted as caused by early-stage/ PAD in asymptomatic diabetic patients. The first investigation of this book provided evidence on the robustness of peak systolic velocity, pulsatility index and resistive index and the weakness of vessel diameter inner to inner in measuring blood flow in asymptomatic diabetic patients with early-stage PAD. Therefore, a decision was made to import peak systolic velocity, pulsatility index and resistive index from the first investigation to compare blood flow between groups in this investigation.

In this investigation thus, the parameters which were to show a significant and meaningful difference between the two groups were to be interpreted as being able to demonstrate the effects of early-stage PAD on lower limb arterial blood flow. This evidence could be utilised in the formation of a new diagnostic pathway for augmenting the screening and quantification of early-stage PAD in diabetic patients using duplex ultrasound.

5.2 Aims

i) To compare blood flow between the diabetic lower limb arteries with early-stage PAD and non-diabetic controls using the ultrasound parameters.
ii) To determine if there were any significant or meaningful differences in, dependent variables (ultrasound parameters) between groups.

5.2.1 Research Questions

i) How do ultrasound parameters compare between diabetic patients with early-stage PAD and non-diabetic controls in the measurement of blood flow?
ii) Are there significant or meaningful differences in ultrasound blood flow parameters between groups?

5.3 Methodology

5.3.1 Design

The principal investigator outlined the design for this Comparative Cohort investigation in section 3.3 of this book. Demographic data collection and stratification of participants with anonymous codes was undertaken by the trained research assistants from the first investigation in-order to minimise selection bias (Paccunni and Wilkins, 2010) through blinding of the principal investigator during this process.

The ultrasound parameters measurements were performed by the principal investigator who was blinded to the archived findings of each coded patient and the robust ultrasound parameters from the first investigation were utilised for lower limb arterial blood flow measurements in this investigation. This control strengthened the rigour of the design and the internal validity of this investigation.

The principal investigator gathered the data for this study over 36 days spanning from the end of May to June 2017, and two patients were booked per day for a scan to allow uncompromised patient care during the gathering of data. The principal investigator performed the ultrasound measurements thrice per each participant and recorded the mean value for each parameter in one measurement session and this minimised measurement error.

5.3.2 Population

The principal investigator drew the sample for this investigation from a population of Black/African diabetic patients attending the diabetic clinic at Mpilo Central Hospital in the city of Bulawayo, Zimbabwe. Black/ African patients formed the majority of the patients attending this clinic and it was feasible to recruit the required sample size through convenience sampling. See section 1.2.1 about the population detail of Zimbabwe. The principal investigator also recruited the control group participants from the staff and students of the National University of Science and Technology through convenience sampling as well.

5.3.3 Sampling

The principal investigator determined the sample size for this investigation through power calculation for the reliability justification of a diagnostic tool and used Schuman's two-sided *t*-test procedure (equation 10a). The principal investigator then calculated the minimum sample size (n) for this investigation as shown in equation 10a;

$$n = \frac{2CV^2 \times (Z_\alpha + Z_\beta)^2}{d^2},$$
10a

Where;

- Coefficient of variation $(CV) = 50\%$, the median intra-individual variability when ultrasound parameters are measured as reported in the literature.

- $Z_\beta = 0.84$, the standard value for normal distribution at power $(\beta) = 80\%$

- $Z_\alpha = 1.96$ the standard value for normal distribution at the level of significance $(\alpha) = 5\%$ i.e.

- $d = 25\%$, the significant difference in the mean value of ultrasound parameters that we expect between health and diseased subjects

- Hence $n = \frac{2CV^2 \times (Z_\alpha + Z_\beta)^2}{d^2} = \frac{2 \times 0.5^2 \times (1.96+0.84)^2}{0.25^2} = 62$ \hspace{2em} 10a

- The principal investigator adjusted for a study dropout of 10% and made the required sample size to be 68 participants (i.e. 34 in the diabetic lower limb arteries group and 34 in the controls).

However, the principal investigator decided to work with a sample of 71 participants who were recruited by the research assistants, with 36 for the non-diabetic control group and 35 for the diabetic group. This sample size was robust enough for justifying the reliability of the ultrasound protocol and was also within the practicalities of the allocated budget for the study. The principal investigator evaluated all hypothesis tests at 5% level of significance ($p \leq 0.05$).

5.3.4 Participants

In this comparative cohort study, the principal investigator compared the lower limb arteries blood flow of a cohort of 35 (49%) asymptomatic diabetic patients (males $n = 10$, females $n = 25$) with early-stage PAD and a control of 36 (51%) non-diabetic participants (males $n = 8$, females $n = 28$) of the same ethnic group (Black/African) and age range (18 -70 years).

The principal investigator outlined the justification for the inclusion and exclusion criteria for the participants for this investigation in section 3.4 of this book. This inclusion criterion included adult participants with early-stage PAD which was objectively confirmed through reactive hyperaemic testing. See section 3.5 in chapter 3 of this book. The principal investigator excluded pregnant participants, as well as smokers and ex-smokers and the justification for this exclusion criteria, is outlined in section 3.4 of this book. The principal investigator outlined the prior preparation of the participants for this investigation in section 3.6 of this book and the recruitment strategy utilised for all the participants in section 3.5 of this book. The research assistants maintained good contact with participants through text messages and telephoning reminding them of their appointment booking as well as their dietary preparations before blood flow measurements. In a bid to confirm participants' adherence to prior dietary preparation instructions, the research assistants instructed the participants to diarise the diet they would have eaten during the three days before the undertaking of blood flow measurements.

The principal investigator highlighted on the information sheets that all the diabetic patients who did not qualify to be categorised as having early-stage PAD were no longer eligible to participate in this investigation but were left to continue their treatment with the physician in the diabetic clinic. Therefore, she instructed the research assistants not to recruit such patients for the sample.

All the participants in both groups provided written informed consent for participation to the principal investigator while the Medical Research Council of Zimbabwe and he Salford University Ethics board approved the study.

5.3.5 Bias from the misclassification of exposure and outcomes.

The principal investigator minimised bias from the misclassification of exposure and outcomes (Paccunni and Wilkins, 2010) by designing prior dietary and medication preparation for the participants in a bid to maintain similar lower limb arterial basal blood flow in participants thus avoiding the masking of the true effects of early-stage PAD. The principal investigator tackled the following external factors in the prior preparation of participants;

i) Effects of recent food intake on blood flow.

ii) Effects of nitrate from consumed nitrate diets,

iii) Effects of meaty diet on creatinine levels in the blood,

iv) Effects of alcohol on blood flow,

v) Effects of diabetes and hypertensive medication before undertaking ultrasound protocol measurements and

vi) Effects of exercise on heart rate, the patients were allowed supine rest of 10 minutes before the undertaking of ultrasound parameters measurements.

In this investigation, bias from the misclassification of exposure and outcomes (Paccunni and Wilkins, 2010) was again minimised through reactive hyperaemic testing of diabetic patients by the physician thus the sample for this investigation was drawn from asymptomatic diabetic participants, with all of them having PAD in the early stages.

Duplex ultrasound which was utilised by the principal investigator to perform the ultrasound measurements for this investigation is an objective test with documented high sensitivity and specificity (Collins et al., 2007; Eiberg et al., 2010) therefore, this minimised measurement error.

5.4 Data collection procedures

5.4.1 Recruitment Plan

In this investigation, 35 diabetic participants with early-stage PAD were recruited by research assistants as they came to Mpilo Central hospital's diabetic clinic during the weekdays when the clinic was open from Tuesday to Thursday. See section 3.5 for the recruitment strategy undertaken until a sample of 35 diabetic patients was reached thus the recruitment of the right lower leg of each diabetic patient for the sake of consistency.

The research assistants recruited the participants for the non-diabetic control group from volunteering staff and students from the National University of Science and Technology, Zimbabwe through a mass e-mail advert which was flown on the University students' and staff members' website by the principal investigator. See section 3.5 for more detail on the recruitment of the sample of 36 non–diabetic control participants.

The Recruitment of the participants for both groups was voluntarily and participants could drop out anytime during the investigation if they so wished without being inconvenienced in any way.

5.4.2 Duplex Ultrasound parameters measurements

The bookings for the second and third investigations were done concurrently by the research assistants three days after the undertaking of the reactive hyperaemic tests. This was done to enable the participants to undergo three days of dietary preparations, absconding alcohol 48 hours before and absconding medication in the morning of the examination day (Section 3.6) before the undertaking of blood tests in the laboratory (section 3.6), Ankle Brachial Index measurements (section 3.7) and duplex ultrasound measurements (section 3.8) by the principal investigator. After the undertaking of the duplex ultrasound measurements for the second investigation by the principal investigator, the research assistants instructed each participant to rest with their gown in the waiting area and assisted them with instructions for the third investigation. See 6.3.2 of this book for more information.

5.5 Statistical analyses

The principal investigator compared all normally distributed demographic data between the two groups using two - samples *t*-test and reported the data as mean (standard deviation [SD]) (Table 5). Additionally, the principal investigator calculated Cohen's *d* effect sizes to determine the magnitude of any differences between the demographic data for these two groups and categorised it according to Cohen, (1988), as *d <0.20 trivial; d = 0.20 - 0.49 small; d = 0.50 - 0.80 medium and d >0.80 large* respectively (Lakens, 2013; Sawilowsky, 2009). The principal investigator compared all non-normal demographic data using the two-sample Wilcoxon's rank-sum test and reported the data as median (interquartile range [IQR]) (Table 5) See section 4.5 for more detail on the justification for normality testing.

The principal investigator documented high blood pressure as the confounding variable between the two samples data to establish its variability amongst the sample exposed to diabetes and the sample not exposed to diabetes using the Chi-square test (Diener-West, 2020).

The first research question of this investigation sought to establish if there was a difference in blood flow between diabetic lower limb arteries with early-stage PAD and non-diabetic controls. Therefore, in a bid to answer the first research question, the principal investigator carried out the analysis for all ultrasound parameters in SPSS (Version 16.0) SPSS, Inc., IL, and USA. The principal investigator then obtained mean values and percentage mean difference values between groups from three within sessions' measurements for each ultrasound parameter which they utilised to calculate within sessions' reliability ICC and the associated 95% confidence interval (CI). Again, the principal investigator classified the ICC values as follows; i) good = 0.60 - 0.74; ii) very good = 0.75 - 0.89 and iii) excellent ≥90 (Koo and Li, 2016). The principal investigator interpreted a significant and meaningful difference in, dependent variables between groups as the ability by ultrasound parameters to demonstrate the effects of early-stage PAD on the blood flow of diabetic patients. This was done in a bid to answer research question 2 of this investigation.

To establish the variability of the ultrasound parameters amongst individuals in each group of participants, the principal investigator calculated the percentage coefficient of variation (%CV) and set the acceptable variability in this investigation at an upper limit of less than 10%CV, thus in comparison to previously established %CV values reporting good reliability (Thomas et al., 2015; Cormack et al., 2008; Sheppard et al., 2011).

5.6 Results

5.6.1 Demographic findings

In a cohort of 71 Black-African participants, 36 (51%) were non-diabetic controls and 35 (49%) were diabetic participants with early-stage PAD. The median for age was significantly higher in diabetic patients compared to non-diabetic patients (Table 6).

The *means (SD)* for Body Mass Index were neither significantly nor meaningfully different between diabetic patients and the non-diabetic controls *(Table 5)*, however, the *median HbA$_{1c}$* levels were significantly higher in diabetic patients when compared to do the non-diabetic controls (Table 6). There were neither significant nor meaningful differences in Ankle Brachial Index between diabetic patients and non-diabetic controls (Table 6).

Table 6: Comparison of subject characteristics between 35 (49%) diabetic patients and 36 (51%) non-diabetic patients where Body Mass Index (BMI) and Ankle Brachial Index (ABI) and Estimated Glomerular Filtration Rate (EGFR did not show a significant or meaningful difference between groups while a significant difference was observed between groups in age and glycated haemoglobin levels (HbA$_{1c}$.)s

Non-normal demographic data

Parameter	Control Median (IQR)	Diabetic Median (IQR)	Two sample t-test p-value	T-test p-value
AGE	37.5 (33 – 54) yrs.	54 (47 – 61) yrs.	0.01	0.01
EGFR	108 (95.5 – 127.5) ml/min/1.73 m^2	112 (96.0 - 126.0) ml/min/1.73 m^2	0.8	0.8
HbA$_{1c}$	5.6 (5.1 – 6.0)%	6.3 (6.0 – 8.0)%	0.0	0.0

Normal demographic data

Parameter	Mean (sd) non-diabetics	Mean (sd) Diabetics	Two sample t-test p-value	Cohen's d effect sizes
BMI	29 (7.0)	29.2 (7.0)	0.7	0.1
ABI	1.1 (0.1)	1.1 (0.1)	0.8	0.1

5.6.2 Association between high blood pressure and diabetic status (Confounding variable)

Table 7 shows that there was a noted significant association between high blood pressure and diabetic participants with early-stage PAD in their lower limb arteries, as reflected by 28 diabetic participants out of 35 had high blood pressure when compared to only 7 non-diabetic participants out of 36 had high blood pressure, ($p < 0.001$).

High Blood Pressure	Status		P-value
	Non-diabetic	Diabetic	
No	29 (81.0%)	7 (20.0%)	
Yes	7 (19.4%)	28 (80.0%)	<0.001
Total	36	35	

5.6.3 The popliteal arteries findings

In the popliteal arteries, the means (SD) for peak systolic velocity, resistive index and pulsatility index was significantly and meaningfully higher in diabetic patients compared to non-diabetic controls (Table 8). Again, peak systolic velocity, pulsatility index and resistive index showed very well to excellent reliability within sessions for diabetic patients and non-diabetic controls and the measurements of all the parameters showed acceptably low variability within sessions for both groups (Table 8).

Table 8 *Descriptive statistics and within sessions reliability of ultrasound parameters in the diabetic and non-diabetic popliteal artery.*

Variable	Mean (SD) diabetic patients	Mean (SD) non-diabetic patients	% mean difference	T-test p-value	Cohen's d effect	ICC within sessions diabetic patients 95% CI	ICC within sessions non-diabetic patients 95% CI	%CV within sessions of diabetic patients	%CV within sessions non-diabetic patients
Peak systolic velocity	73.0 (10.3) cm/s	56.3 (5.3) cm/s	16.2%	<0.0001	2.0	1.0 (1.0 – 1.0)	1.0 (1.0 – 1.0)	1.1%	0.3%
Pulsatility index	8.2 (2.3)	9.0 (3.0)	0.4%	0.5	0.2	1.0 (1.0 – 1.0)	1.0 (1.0 – 1.0)	9.0%	5.4%
Resistive index	1.1 (0.1)	1.0 (0.1)	6.1%	<0.001	1.0	0.9 (0.7 – 1.0)	0.7 (0.5 – 0.8)	7.0%	2.3%

SD = standard deviation; ICC = intraclass correlation coefficient; %CV = percentage coefficient of variation; %mean difference = percentage mean difference

5.6.4 Anterior tibial artery (ATA) findings

In the anterior tibial arteries, the means (ds) for peak systolic velocity, pulsatility index and the resistive index was significantly and meaningfully higher in diabetic patients compared to non-diabetic patients (Table 9). Again, peak systolic velocity, pulsatility index and resistive index showed good to excellent reliability within sessions for all the groups and acceptably low variability was noted in the measurements of all the parameters in both groups except in pulsatility index for the diabetic patients (Table 9).

Table 9 Descriptive statistics and within sessions reliability of ultrasound parameters in the diabetic and non-diabetic anterior tibial arteries.

Variable	Mean(SD) diabetic patients	Mean (SD) non-diabetic patients	% mean difference	T-test p-value	Cohen's d effect sizes	ICC within sessions diabetic patients 95% CI	ICC within sessions non-diabetic patients 95% CI	%CV within sessions diabetic patients	%CV within sessions non-diabetic patients
Peak systolic velocity	47.0 (9.0) cm/s	40.0 (7.2) cm/s	17.0 %	<0.001	0.8	1.0 (1.0 - 1.0)	1.0 (1.0 - 1.0)	1.7%	0.7%
Pulsatility index	8.0 (2.2)	7.0 (2.0)	12.0%	<0.001	0.4	0.9 (0.8 - 1.0)	1.0 (1.0 - 1.0)	**11.1%**	4.5%
Resistive index	1.1 (0.1)	1.0 (0.1)	6.0%	<0.001	0.6	0.7 (0.5 - 0.8)	0.7 (0.4 - 0.8)	5.2%	3.0%

SD = standard deviation; ICC = intraclass correlation coefficient; %CV = percentage coefficient of variation; SDD = smallest detectable difference; SEM = standard error of measurement

5.6.5 Posterior tibial artery (PTA) findings

In the posterior tibial arteries, the means (SD) for peak systolic velocity and the resistive index was significantly and meaningfully higher in diabetic patients compared to non-diabetic patients, other than pulsatility index (Table10). Again, peak systolic velocity, pulsatility index and resistive index showed good to excellent within sessions reliability in both groups and the variability amongst measurements of all parameters in both groups was acceptable (Table 10).

Table 10 Descriptive statistics and within sessions reliability of ultrasound parameters in the diabetic and non-diabetic posterior tibial artery.

Variable	Mean (SD) diabetic patients	Mean (SD) non-diabetic patients	% Mean Difference	T-test p-value	Cohen's d effect sizes	ICC within sessions of diabetic patients 95% CI	ICC within sessions non-diabetic patients 95% CI	%CV within sessions of diabetic patients	%CV within sessions no n-diabetic patients
Peak systolic velocity	44.0 (12.0) cm/s	41.0 (8.0) cm/s	9.0%	0.01	0.3	1.0 (1.0 - 1.0)	1.0 (1.0 - 1.0)	2.0%	0.6%
Pulsatility index	7.0 (5.1)	7.0 (2.0)	3.0%	0.7	0.1	1.0 (1.0 - 1.0)	1.0 (0.9 - 1.0)	10.0%	4.3%
Resistive index	1.1 (0.2)	1.0 (0.1)	5.1%	<0.001	0.4	0.7 (0.5 - 0.85)	0.8 (0.7 - 0.9)	8.0%	3.0%

SD = standard deviation; ICC = intraclass correlation coefficient; %CV = percentage coefficient of variation; %mean difference = percentage mean difference

5.7 Discussion

5.7.1 Duplex ultrasound parameters.

In this investigation, the ultrasound parameters consisting of peak systolic velocity, resistive index and pulsatility index were significantly and meaningfully higher ($P < 0.001$; $d \geq 0.3$), in diabetic patients compared to non-diabetic controls except for pulsatility index of the posterior tibial arteries ($P = 0.7$; $d = 0.1$). All the ultrasound parameters showed good ($ICC \geq 0.7$; $0.5 - 0.9$, 95% CI) to excellent ($ICC \leq 1.0$; $1.0 - 1.0$, 95% CI) within sessions reliability as well as acceptable variability (<10% CV) within groups except pulsatility index of the anterior tibial arteries for diabetic patients (11.1%CV) (Tables 8; 9; 10). These findings were in line with the research question for this investigation which sought to determine if the ultrasound parameters could show a difference in blood flow between the diabetic lower limb arteries with early-stage (asymptomatic) PAD and the non-diabetic controls. A Significant and meaningful difference in blood flow between the two groups was interpreted as the ability to demonstrate the effects of early-stage PAD on the lower limb blood flow of diabetic patients while the non-significant and non-meaningful difference in blood flow between the two groups was interpreted as an inability to demonstrate the effects of early-stage PAD on the lower limb blood flow of diabetic patients. The findings of this investigation showed peak systolic and resistive index as robust ultrasound parameters able to detect a difference in blood flow between diabetic patients with early-stage (asymptomatic) PAD and non-diabetic controls. Thus, peak systolic velocity and resistive index were concluded as the ones able to demonstrate the effects of early-stage PAD on the lower limb blood flow of diabetic patients with the exclusion of the pulsatility index.

In the first investigation with a smaller sample size (n = 10), within sessions reliability ranged from very good (ICC ≥ 0.8; $0.6 - 0.9$, 95% CI) to excellent (ICC

≤1.0; 1.0 – 1.0, 95%CI) with a %CV of less or equal to 5.6%. Similarly, in this investigation having a larger sample size (n = 35 diabetic patients; n = 36 non-diabetic patients) within sessions reliability ranged from good (ICC ≥ 0.7; 0.5 – 0.9, 95% CI) to excellent (ICC ≤1.0; 1.0 – 1.0. 95%CI) with a %CV of less than 10%. These findings reflected that the ultrasound parameters were robust in measuring blood flow in the lower limbs of diabetic patients with early-stage PAD as well as in the non-diabetic controls.

Most of the ultrasound parameters showed a high mean percentage difference (less or equal to 16%) between groups compared to the Smallest Detectable Difference (9.2%) of individual successive measurements done in the first investigation for the popliteal arteries and anterior tibial arteries. This reflected that the change in blood flow seen in diabetic patients with early-stage PAD in the popliteal arteries and anterior tibial arteries was of clinical significance and would call for a change in the management of the diabetic patients (Tables 8 and 9).

In the posterior tibial arteries for this investigation, the ultrasound parameters showed smaller values for the mean percentage difference (less or equal to 8.5%) between groups compared to the Smallest detectable difference (7.7%) from successive individual measurements in the first investigation thus, reflecting that the blood flow changes observed in the posterior tibial artery due to early-stage PAD were not clinically significant.

A study by Zhang et al., (2013) reported that resistive index of the acral finger was significantly higher (p <0.001) in diabetic patients with late-stage (symptomatic) PAD compared to non-diabetic controls. Similarly, their results also reflected that RI in diabetic patients became even higher as the duration of diabetes mellitus increased (P <0.01). Jansen, (2005) also showed that pulsatility index was reduced in late-stage PAD, their findings showed that a pulsatility index of <1.2 indicated critical limb ischaemia with a sensitivity of 0.9 and a specificity of 0.6 while Ankle Brachial Index of less than 0.9 showed a sensitivity of 0.7 and a specificity of 0.4. However, the findings of Jansen, (2005) were in diabetic patients with late-stage (symptomatic) PAD and this scenario peak systolic velocity reduced while end-diastolic velocity was mostly absent due to increasing resistance to blood flow thus resulting in a smaller value of pulsatility index as depicted by the formula for pulsatility index in equation 1 chapter 2. Therefore the findings of these prior studies all provided evidence on the utilisation of ultrasound parameters to detect and grade late-stage (symptomatic) PAD.

The findings of this investigation showed different mean values for ultrasound parameters in the lower limb blood flow of Zimbabwean Black/African diabetic patients with early-stage PAD and non-diabetic controls when compared to prior published range values of healthy individuals and diabetic patients with late-stage PAD. In this investigation, the mean value for peak systolic velocity in the popliteal arteries of diabetic patients with early-stage PAD was 72.9 ± 10.3 cm/s while prior evidence (Hodgkiss-Harlow and Bandyk, 2014; Chavhan et al, 2008), has shown a peak systolic velocity of greater than 180 cm/s elicited in arterial stenosis of greater or equal to 50%. This confirmed that the sample participants for this investigation could have been having arterial stenosis of way less than 50% stenosis but the ultrasound parameters still managed to demonstrate the effects of early-stage PAD in the blood flow of these diabetic patients. Therefore, this evidence justifies the need to utilise duplex ultrasound parameters to enhance screening and quantification of early-stage PAD in asymptomatic diabetic patients alongside the prior recommended Ankle Brachial Index.

In this investigation, the mean value for peak systolic velocity in the popliteal arteries of non-diabetic controls was lower (55.3 ± 3 cm/s) compared to prior published mean normal value for other healthy populations (68 ± 1 cm/s). These different values for blood flow shown by peak systolic velocity maybe be due to different ethnicities, lifestyles or diets of the sample populations of participants in the different studies (Sanna et al., 2011). In their study, Sanna et al., (2011) also noted that the epidemiology of PAD was not homogenous amongst different ethnic populations with diverse lifestyles and diets.

Prior evidence (Gerhard-Herman et al, 2006; Hodgkiss-Harlow and Bandyk, 2014) has shown the normal ranges for the peak systolic velocity of tibial arteries in healthy individuals as 55 ± 1 cm/s while this investigation findings in non-diabetic controls showed a lower mean peak systolic velocity of the anterior tibial arteries (40.0 ± 7.2 cm/s) and the mean peak systolic velocity for the posterior tibial arteries was lower as well (40.6 ± 8.0 cm/s).

The pulsatility index for the popliteal arteries in healthy individuals in prior studies was shown as greater than 8 (Gerhard-Herman et al, 2006; Hodgkiss-Harlow and Bandyk, 2014) while in this investigation the mean pulsatility index value for the non-diabetic controls was lower and shown as (6.9 ± 2.1).

5.7.2 Ankle Brachial Index (ABI)

The principal investigator utilised Ankle-Brachial index as a complementary parallel test alongside the ultrasound protocol parameters to detect early-stage PAD in asymptomatic diabetic patients (Rooke et al., 2011; Gerhard-Herman et al., 2016; Norgren et al., 2007; Carthy 2013). The test has been recommended in practice guidelines to screen and quantify early stage (symptomatic) PAD in prior studies undertaken in other populations, and Ankle Brachial Index values less or equal to 0.9 reflect PAD in the lower limb arteries (Rooke et al., 2011; Gerhard-Herman et al., 2016; Norgren et al., 2007; Carthy 2013).

In this investigation, there was no significant difference, ($P > 0.05$) in the values for Ankle Brachial Index between the groups thus Ankle Brachial Index was a weaker test in demonstrating early stage (asymptomatic) PAD in diabetic patients while ultrasound parameters including peak systolic velocity and resistive index demonstrated the effects of early-stage PAD in the blood flow of participants with Ankle Brachial Index values greater than 0.9 (Table 6).

Late-stage PAD results in pressure reduction in the ankle arteries while the upper arm arteries will still be yet unaffected, thus resulting in a lower value for Ankle Brachial Index in such patients. However, the case is not true in early-stage (asymptomatic) PAD because pressure reduction will not yet be taking place in the ankle arteries, thus when they get divided by the unaffected upper arms pressure the result would reflect normal values of Ankle Brachial Index of around 1. See section 2.1.4 for more information on how the Ankle Brachial Index is calculated.

5.7.3 Confounding variables

In this investigation, the noted confounding variable was high blood pressure and findings of this investigation showed a positive correlative relationship between diabetes and medical history of high blood pressure (Table 7).

5.7.4 Strengths and Limitations

The strength of this investigation was that it was carried out under controlled settings which were put in place by the principal investigator to limit performance, recall, selection and misclassification of exposure and outcomes bias as well as measurement error. This investigation aimed to compare ultrasound parameters measurements of blood flow between the groups which were incomparable conditions when the measurements were taken, such that the lapse period of one month over which the data was gathered by the principal investigator did not matter even if it could have allowed the accumulation of a thicker plaque than initial values at the beginning of the month since the investigation was not aimed at investigating any changes in blood flow with time.

5.7.5 Internal and external validity

This investigation had good internal validity since principal investigator put in place a rigorous inclusion and exclusion criteria, and recruitment strategy for the sample which minimised the effects of bias. The simple random sampling which was utilised by the research assistants during recruitment of the study sample allowed a fair chance of recruitment of all participants while this process was blinded to the principal investigator, who held knowledge of the exposure and outcomes of the study. The principal investigator was also blinded during the collection and analysis of data.

In this investigation, the variables considered were exposure to diabetes in early stages or non-exposure to diabetes in the participants while the outcome measured was blood flow in the lower limb arteries and the principal investigator conducted this investigation under idealised controlled measures such that the findings of this investigation were representative of the true association between exposure and expected outcome and thus could be generalised to the population of Zimbabwean Black/African asymptomatic diabetic patients with early-stage PAD. However, the findings of this investigation could not conclude generalisability to other populations resident in Zimbabwe besides Black/Africans due to lack of heterogeneity in the sample.

The principal investigator stratified the confounding variable of high blood pressure amongst the participants of both groups and established its correlation with both groups.

5.8 Conclusions

There were significant and meaningful differences between the lower limb blood flow of diabetic patients with early-stage PAD and non-diabetic controls as determined by peak systolic velocity and resistive index with diabetic patients exhibiting higher values compared to controls except pulsatility index. Therefore, the principal investigator concluded that peak systolic velocity and resistive index were capable of demonstrating the effects of early-stage PAD on the blood flow of asymptomatic diabetic patients while pulsatility index was a weaker parameter due to more measurement errors in the anterior tibial arteries and posterior tibial arteries.

5.9 Decision making

The principal investigator then decided to continue the assessment of peak systolic velocity and resistive index from this investigation to the third investigation of this book due to the robustness they demonstrated with the exclusion of pulsatility Index due to the demonstrated high percentage coefficient of variation. However, the principal investigator will assess the anterior tibial arteries and posterior tibial arteries with peak systolic velocity and the resistive index separately in post-doctoral work to reduce error in timing if two arterial segments were to be assessed in the same time slot for blood flow effects which quickly wan off. The principal investigator will also assess RI later in the postdoctoral work in a bid to reduce the number of parameters to be assessed in the third investigation thus allowing a more focussed assessment of peak systolic velocity.

5.10 Recommendations

In this in the investigation, the principal investigator made the following recommendations;

i) Duplex ultrasound parameters including peak systolic velocity and resistive index may be utilised to screen and quantify effects of early-stage (asymptomatic) PAD on the blood flow of diabetic patients with an Ankle Brachial Index value of greater than 0.90.

ii) Ankle Brachial Index findings for screening and quantifying early-stage PAD may be enhanced with duplex ultrasound parameters such as peak systolic velocity and resistive index.

iii) All patients at risk for PAD may need mandatory lower limb blood flow assessment with ultrasound parameters such as peak systolic velocity and resistive index while still in the secondary care of the Zimbabwean health delivery system.

5.11 Implications of the second investigation

The principal investigator deducted the implications of this investigation as that duplex ultrasound parameters including peak systolic velocity and resistive index were robust in demonstrating the effects of early-stage PAD on the lower limb blood flow of diabetic patients. Therefore, all diabetic patients in secondary care of the Zimbabwean health delivery system need to be screened with these parameters to enable enhanced quantification of early-stage PAD to prompt earlier introduction of therapy.

Chapter 6 - Third investigation
Abstract
Acute effects of beetroot juice on blood flow and blood pressure in diabetic patients with early-stage PAD compared to non-diabetic controls.

Keywords: *peripheral arterial disease, nitrite, nitric oxide, peak systolic velocity, systolic blood pressure, diastolic blood pressure.*

Objective: To determine the acute effects of beetroot juice ingestion on blood flow and blood pressure in diabetic patients with early-stage PAD compared to non-diabetic controls.

Methods: A quasi-experimental cohort study of lower limb blood flow in 35 Black-African diabetic patients and 36 non-diabetic controls *who were imported from the second investigation)*. PSV, systolic blood pressure (SBP) and diastolic blood pressure (DBP) were utilised to assess blood flow in the popliteal arteries (PA), 90 minutes, 150 minutes, and 210 minutes-post-ingestion of beetroot juice both between and within groups. A two-way analysis of variance and a Benferroni test was performed to compare the two groups across 4-time points after the intake of beetroot juice. One sample and two-sample t-tests with Cohen's d effects sizes were performed to determine whether any changes in dependant variables were significant and meaningful within groups and between groups respectively.

Results: Within groups, PSV, SBP and DBP reduced significantly and meaningfully during baseline to 90 minutes and 150 minutes-210 minutes time points *(P ≤0.02; d ≤1.70)*. However, no significant /meaningful change *(P ≤0.9; d ≤0.29)* occurred in PSV, SBP and DBP during the 90 minutes to 150 minutes time point. Between groups, PSV and DBP were significantly and meaningfully higher *(P ≤0.04; d ≤1.95)* in diabetic patients at baseline. However, at 90 minutes and 150 minutes PSV remained higher in diabetic patients *(P ≤0.04; d ≤1.30)* unlike SBP *(P ≤0.8); d ≤0.34)*. At 210 minutes, PSV and SBP did not change significantly or meaningfully *(P ≤0.59; d ≤0.18)* while DBP showed no significant or meaningful difference *(P ≤0.7; d ≤0.33)* between the groups at all the time points. The combined group effects were significant for PSV *(diff ≤ 20.0 cm/s; P <0.0001)* across all the time points except between 90 minutes to 150 minutes *(diff = 0.4cm/s; P = 1.0)* The combined group effects were significant for SBP *(diff ≤22.01mmHg; P <0.0001)* amongst all the time points except 90 minutes to 150 minutes time point *(diff = 1.2 mmHg; P = 1.00)* and finally the combined group effects for DBP were significant and meaningful *(diff ≤13.4 mmHg; P <0.0001)* amongst all the time points except 90 minutes to 150 minutes *(diff = 1.34 mmHg; P = 1.00)* after beetroot juice ingestions.

Conclusions: The acute effects of beetroot juice on the blood flow of the popliteal artery were reflected as lowered PSV, SBP and DBP during the 150-210 minutes time point.

Correspondence to: Josephine S Tityiwe, National University of Science and Technology, Radiography, Department, Corner Cecil/Gwanda Road, P. O. Box AC 939 Ascot, Bulawayo, Zimbabwe. Email: josephine.tityiwe@nust.ac.zw/ J.S.Tityiwe@edu.salford.ac.uk

6.1 Introduction

Type 2 Diabetes mellitus is a risk factor for cardiovascular complications which include PAD and microvascular complications which include retinopathy, nephropathy, cerebrovascular disease erectile dysfunction to mention a few. This is mainly due to atherosclerosis/plaque build-up which occurs in the endothelium of the blood vessels of these diabetic patients (Steinberg, 2009; Steinberg and Wizturn, 2010). Chronically as atherosclerotic lesions are progressively deposited in the lumen of arteries in diabetic patients the process then becomes PAD and usually starts manifesting significantly in small diameter lower limb arteries below the knees. This gradual arterial stenosis due to plaque build-up in the endothelium manifests following endothelial cells injury by diabetes. This injury of the endothelium impairs the nitric oxide-L-arginine pathway thus reducing the bioavailability of nitric oxide which forms the anti-oxidation defence system to clear away reactive oxygen species, low-density lipoproteins and free radicals which are mostly produced during a host of defence and immunologic reactions by activated macrophages, preventing them from continually aggregating in the endothelium (Steinberg, 2009; Steinberg and Wizturn, 2010). This altered L-arginine-nitric oxide pathway and impaired nitric oxide bioavailability when uncontrolled it contributes to an acceleration of complications such as PAD, Hypertension and Cardiovascular diseases (Umans and Levi, 1995; Davignon and Ganz, 2004; Bahadoran et al., 2015; Siervo et al., 2013).

The UK and USA guidelines on adult Diabetes management outline the prescription of Aspirin/Clopidogrel as antiplatelet therapy, besides advising on smoking cessation, healthy eating of foods with high fibre, and foods with low glycaemic index sources of carbohydrate, increasing physical activity and exercise and self-monitored feet care (Eisenstein et al., 2017; Type 2 Diabetes in adults: management (NG 28), NICE, 2015). Diets containing natural inorganic nitrate have were found to be exogenous sources for the much-needed nitric oxide in patients suffering from highly inflammatory and oxidative diseases like Type 2 diabetes and evidence has shown that these diets rich in inorganic nitrate are associated with inhibition of platelet aggregation, preservation, and improvement of endothelial dysfunction which may be caused by diabetes in the arterial walls, these include beetroot, usually in the form of a juice, green leafy vegetables such as spinach, rocket and lettuce were also found to contain large sources of inorganic nitrate (Clements et al., 2014; Lundberg et al., 2008; Doel et al., 2005; Hyde et al., 2014). Prior evidence has proven beetroot juice as a popular vasodilator and has been used successfully in the treatment and reduction of blood pressure, in subjects with cardiovascular disease and Type 2 Diabetes as well (Clifford et al., 2015; Siervo et al., 2013; Bahadoran et al., 2015; Gilchrist et al., 2013; Kenjale et al., 2011), Therefore, it was justifiable to administer beetroot juice to diabetic patients with early-stage PAD in this investigation to assess its effects on the lower limb blood flow with ultrasound peak systolic velocity and blood pressure.

Nitric oxide gas is produced endogenously from the amino acid L-arginine pathway by three isoforms of nitric oxide synthases in the endothelium of blood vessels, and it is useful as an anti-oxidation defence system and an antiplatelet thus inhibiting the acceleration of atherosclerosis (Stamler et al., 1989; Steinberg, 2009, Steinberg and Wizturn, 2010, Cooke, 1996; Stamler, 1989). Beetroot contains inorganic nitrate as the main bioactive component behind the reduction of blood pressure (Webb et al., 2008) and endurance exercise interactions (Vanhatalo et al., 2011) as well. In another study, Gilchrist et al., (2014), administered Beetroot juice (nitrate content 7.5 mmol) versus beetroot juice placebo (nitrate content 0.002 mmol) to type 2 diabetic patients and noted a significant improvement in simple reaction time *(P <0.05)* in individuals who had blindly ingested beetroot juice with 7.5 mmol inorganic nitrate content compared to those who had blindly ingested placebo beetroot juice, thus strengthening the evidence that inorganic nitrate was the main bioactive component responsible for the noted change.

Following oral consumption of foods rich in inorganic nitrate such as beetroot juice, the nitrate is quickly absorbed in the stomach, duodenum and jejunum and availed in the circulation. Later about 25% is excreted in the oral cavity where commensal bacteria anaerobes (via nitrate reductive enzymes) mainly found under the back of the tongue bio-activate nitrate and reduce it to nitrite in saliva (the entero-salivary circulation) and about 75% of the nitrate is excreted via kidneys (Kapil et al., 2010; Vanhatalo et al., 2010). When this nitrite is swallowed into the acidic stomach, some of it is bio-activated into nitric oxide then both the nitric oxide and nitrite are rapidly absorbed into the circulation peaking this bioavailability from 2.5 – 3 hrs (Kapil et al., 2010; Vanhatalo et al., 2010; Webb et al., 2008).

The main purpose of the availed nitric oxide is to maintain endothelial function in the inner walls of the arteries thus maintaining vascular homeostasis through maintaining the oxidative defence system, platelet function, vascular tone and the delicate balance between vasodilation and vasoconstriction (Clifford et al., 2015; Hobbs et al., 2012; Davignon and Ganz, 2004), thus a depletion in nitric oxide availability has been concluded as the main cause of endothelial dysfunction, a risk factor of cardiovascular disorders and in the pathogenesis of hypertension and atherosclerosis (Lidder et al., 2013; Joris and Mensik, 2013). Beetroot juice has been well researched and is being considered as a promising therapy in a range of clinical pathologies associated with oxidative stress and inflammation (Clifford et al., 2015), Being a source of inorganic nitrate, ingestion of Beetroot juice increases the bioavailability of nitric oxide to manage these pathologies associated with diminished nitric oxide availability, such as diabetes, hypertension, dyslipidaemia to mention a few, thus diminishing the rate of atherosclerosis (Kapil, 2010; Clements et al., 2014; Clifford et al., 2015; Kannady et al., 2012), and in all these studies no known adverse reactions were encountered besides short term effects such as beeturia, red stools, reduction in blood pressure and gastrointestinal discomfort

(Kenjale et al., 2011, Webb et al., 2008, Vanhatalo et al., 2010; Bahadoran et al., 2015; Gilchrist et al., 2013).

Zimbabwe is experiencing the same chronic global problem of the prevalence of diabetes mellitus in its population as well the increased death risk from the complications of diabetes such as PAD in these patients (Parirenyatwa and Gwinji, 2016; Hakim et al., 2005). There was no prior evidence establishing the acute effects of beetroot juice ingestion on blood flow in the lower limbs of diabetic patients with early-stage PAD and non-diabetic controls using ultrasound during the writing up of this book. This investigation, therefore, aimed to provide justifying evidence to fill this existing gap in the literature by utilising duplex ultrasound peak systolic velocity alongside systolic blood pressure and diastolic blood pressure. The justification for utilising peak systolic velocity in this investigation was because its robustness in measuring lower limb blood flow was established in the first investigation of this book and its ability to demonstrate the effects of early-stage/asymptomatic PAD on the lower limb blood flow of diabetic patients was also established in the second investigation of this book.

In this investigation, the aim was to determine if there were detectable acute effects in blood flow post beetroot juice ingestion in diabetic lower limb arteries with early-stage PAD and the non-diabetic controls using peak systolic velocity, systolic blood pressure and diastolic blood pressure. Evidence from this investigation may be used in the formation of an affordable and cheap therapeutic pathway for managing early-stage PAD in diabetic patients.

6.2 Aim

i) To determine the acute effects of beetroot juice ingestion on blood flow within and between the diabetic lower limb arteries with early-stage PAD and non-diabetic controls using peak systolic velocity and blood pressure.

6.2.1 Research questions

i) Is there a change in the blood flow of non-diabetic lower limb arteries after beetroot juice ingestion as determined by peak systolic velocity and blood pressure (at 90minutes; 150 minutes and 210 minutes)?

ii) Is there a change in the blood flow of diabetic lower limb arteries after beetroot juice ingestion as determined by peak systolic velocity and blood pressure (at 90 minutes; 150 minutes and 210 minutes)?

iii) Is there a difference in the blood flow changes between non-diabetic and diabetic lower limb arteries after beetroot juice ingestion as determined by peak systolic velocity and blood pressure?

6.3 Methodology

6.3.1 Design

The design for this quasi-experimental investigation is outlined in section 3.3 of this book. This investigation was a continuation of the second investigation and the principal investigator carried it out soon after each participant had completed the measurements for the second investigation. The principal investigator imported the socio-demographic history and Ankle-brachial Index values from the second investigation into this investigation. Again, the principal investigator imported the duplex ultrasound findings for peak systolic velocity of the popliteal artery for each participant from the second investigation as basal blood flow findings in this investigation. However, the principal investigator also assessed the basal systolic and diastolic blood pressure for each participant for this investigation before they were administered beetroot juice for ingestion.

Prior evidence has shown beetroot juice as effective in reducing blood pressure, (Clifford et al., 2015; Gilchrist et al., 2013; Bahadoran et al., 2015; Kenjale et al., 2011; Vanhatalo et al., 2010; Webb et al., 2008), thus the principal investigator instructed the patients not to take blood pressure medications in the morning of the examination day to avoid masking the true effects of beetroot juice on blood pressure. However, the principal investigator instructed the participants to take their blood pressure medications after undertaking the last blood pressure measurement at 210 minutes after ingesting beetroot juice only if their blood pressure did not fall in the normal range of

$\frac{120-130}{80-90}$ mmHg or slightly lower. 9

All the participants in both groups had already provided written informed consent forms for participation which were approved by the Medical Research Council of Zimbabwe and the Salford University Ethics board to the principal investigator during the undertaking of the second investigation.

6.3.2 Population and Sampling

The principal investigator imported the sample for both groups for this investigation from the second investigation and the criteria for having early-stage PAD was still the same as outlined in section 5.3.4 of chapter 5 of this book. In this case, transfer bias from the second investigation to this investigation was minimised since each participant simply continued from the second into this investigation on the same day before being dismissed to go home.

6.3.3 Participants

The participants of this investigation were imported from the second investigation by the principal investigator. See section 5.3.4 chapter 5 of book for more detail on the demographic data and sections 3.4 and 5.3.5 for the outlined justification for the inclusion and exclusion criteria utilised for this investigation.

6.4 Data collection procedures

6.4.1 Body Mass Index measurements

The Body Mass Index and Ankle Brachial Index measurements which were performed in the second investigation were imported into this investigation. See section 4.4 of chapter 4 and section 3.7 of chapter 3 of this book for more detail.

6.4.2 Duplex Ultrasound and Blood pressure measurements

After the completion of the measurements for the second investigation, each participant continued into this investigation. The diabetic clinic-based physician was on stand by for the monitoring of any anaphylactic reactions to beetroot juice ingestion which could have been elicited by the participants and the principal investigator had in place the correct protocol of management with the Medical Research Council of Zimbabwe to cater for any adverse reactions taking place in any participants following ingestion of the beetroot juice intervention. See Appendix J for more detail on the Medical Research Council of Zimbabwe adverse reactions form.

The research assistants instructed each participant to relax on the examination bed for about 10 minutes in a supine position to allow a stable heart rate for a stable basal blood flow in the participants' lower limbs arteries.

The principal investigator then measured the participants' blood pressure at rest from the non-dependent upper arm at a similar position for each participant with an automated blood pressure machine (CareVue, Shenzhen, China), and recorded the basal systolic and diastolic blood pressure values while the research assistants later collated the blood pressure readings with each participant's anonymous code.

Concurrently the blood flow results for peak systolic velocity from the second investigation (Section 5.6.3 of in chapter 5) were collated as the baseline readings for each participant in this investigation by the research assistants.

After completion of basal blood pressure, the research assistants instructed each participant to sit in the waiting area and administered 500 ml of beetroot juice (7.38 mmol beetroot juice nitrate) orally to each of them. See Figure 1 in chapter 1 of this book for the type of beetroot juice administered in this investigation. However, the principal investigator allowed the diabetic patients to take their medication together with beetroot juice and the justification for this is outlined in section 3.6 of this book.

The research assistants instructed each participant to relax for the initial 80 minutes to allow for the digestion and processing of beetroot juice in the stomach (Kapil et al, 2010; Vanhatalo et al, 2010). After the initial 80 minutes of relaxing following beetroot juice ingestion, the research assistants helped each participant back on the couch and allowed them another 10 minutes supine rest on the couch to enable the participants to achieve a stable heart rate. The principal investigator then started measuring the participants' blood pressure in the non-dependant arm upper followed by blood flow measurements in the right lower limb using peak systolic velocity at 90 minutes, 150 minutes and 210 minutes post beetroot juice intake respectively.

Blood flow and blood pressure measurements were started at 90 minutes after beetroot juice ingestions to allow the capturing of the earlier effects of beetroot juice on blood flow even though prior evidence has shown that presumed vasodilation from orally administered beetroot juice occurred after about 180 minutes (Kapil et al, 2010; Vanhatalo et al, 2010). A pre-set alarm was put in place with the respective timings by the research assistants to enable effective and smooth flow of timing across the three-time points after beetroot juice intake.

The same principal investigator from the first and second investigations measured the blood flow and the blood pressure in this investigation and this minimised performance bias. For each participant, the principal investigator recorded the values for peak systolic velocity measurements in the archives of the duplex ultrasound machine for each time slot thus at 90 minutes, 150 minutes and finally at 210 minutes under the anonymised codes for each participant. Later the research assistants collated the anonymised coded peak systolic velocity measurements for each patient with their blood pressure measurements and demographic data in Microsoft Excel sheets.

After the principal investigator measured and recorded the blood pressure for each participant at 210 minutes post beetroot juice ingestion, and if the blood pressure was found to be within the normal range values (Equation 9; Eisenstein et al., 2017) then the principal investigator advised the participant not to take their blood pressure reducing medications on that day but to resume on the following day to avoid reducing the blood pressure below the normal range.

The scanning technique utilised by the principal investigator to assess the popliteal arteries in this investigation is outlined in section 3.8 of chapter 3 of this book.

After the all the measurements were completed, the research assistants gave each participant a refreshment of 100% pure juice and low sugar biscuit and instructed the participants to relax in the ultrasound department for about 20 minutes before dismissing them home.

6.5 Statistical analyses

The principal investigator imported the demographic data which was analysed from the second investigation into this investigation. See section 5.6 for more detail on the statistical analysis of demographic data which was done in the second investigation (Table 5).

The principal investigator performed a two-way analysis of variance (ANOVA) (2 x 4; group x time) and post - hoc analysis using the Benferroni test to compare the two groups thus diabetic patients and non-diabetic controls across 4-time points enabling the comparison of combined groups effects at specific time points after the ingestion of beetroot juice. This was undertaken by the principal investigator in a bid to answer research question three which sought to determine if there was a difference in blood flow between the two groups with time as indicated by dependent variables (peak systolic velocity and blood pressure). The principal investigator performed two samples *t*-test and Cohen's *d* effect sizes to compare the means of dependent variables between groups at each specific time point to establish if these differences were significant and meaningful and an a priori alpha was set at 0.05 level of significance.

Again, the principal investigator performed one-sample *t*-test and Cohen's d effect sizes to compare the means of dependent variables within each group between specific time points within each group and Cohen's *d* effect sizes were performed to establish if these differences were significant and meaningful. One sample *t*-test and two samples *t*-test were performed to try and answer research questions 1 and 2 which sought to determine any change in blood flow within groups and between groups at specific time points respectively as determined by the dependent variables (peak systolic velocity and blood pressure) after beetroot juice ingestion. See section 5.5 for more detail on the effect sizes which were set for this investigation.

6.6 Results

6.6.1 Demographic findings

In a cohort of 71 Black-African participants, 36 (51%) were non-diabetic controls and 35 (49%) were diabetic participants with early-stage PAD. Since the principal investigator imported the participants for this investigation from the second investigation, therefore the demographic findings were similarly the same as outlined in section 5.6.1 table 6.

6.6.2 Combined groups peak systolic velocity changes after beetroot juice ingestion at specific time points.

Combined group effects for peak systolic velocity showed a significant change *(diff ≤ 12.3 cm/s; P ≤0.0001)* between the baseline and 90 minutes time point, the baseline and 150 minutes time point *(diff; 14.0 cm/s; P ≤0.0001)*, the baseline and 210 minutes time point *(diff = 20.0 cm/s; P ≤0.0001)* and the 150 minutes and 210 minutes time point *(diff = 6.0 cm/s; P <0.0001)*. However there was no significant change in peak systolic velocity *(diff = 0.4cm/s; P = 1.00)* between the 90 minutes and 150 minutes time point after beetroot juice ingestions (table 11).

Table 11 Combined groups' peak systolic velocity changes after beetroot juice ingestion at specific time points (Benferroni).

	baseline	90 minutes	150 minutes
90 minutes	-12.3 cm/s (diff) $P = 0.000$		
150 minutes	-14.0 cm/s (diff) $P = 0.000$	-2.0 cm/s (diff) $P = 1.000$	
210 minutes	-20.0 cm/s (diff) $P = 0.000$	-8.0 cm/s (diff) $P = 0.000$	-6.0 cm/s (diff) $P = 0.000$
Diff = mean difference; p = value			

6.6.3 Peak systolic velocity comparisons between groups at specific time points.

Between groups, peak systolic velocity was significantly and meaningfully higher (P <0.0001; d = 1.95) in diabetic patients (73.0 ± 11.0 cm/s) compared to non-diabetic patients (56.3 ± 5.3 cm/s) basally. After beetroot juice ingestions at 90 minutes peak systolic velocity was again significantly and meaningfully higher (P <0.0001; d = 1.30) in diabetic patients (57.0 ± 8.1 cm/s) compared to non-diabetic patients (48.0 ± 5.2 cm/s). At 150 minutes peak systolic velocity was still significantly and meaningfully higher (P <0.0001; d = 1.10) in diabetic patients (54.1 ± 8.0 cm/s) compared to non-diabetic patients (47.0 ± 5.0 cm/s). However, at 210 minutes there was neither a significant nor meaningful difference (P = 0.4; d = 0.18) in peak systolic velocity between diabetic patients (45.2 ± 9.0 cm/s) compared to non-diabetic patients (44.0 ± 4.0 cm/s) (Table 12 ; Figure 12).

Table 12 Comparison of peak systolic velocity changes between groups at specific time points

Parameter	Mean (sd) Non-diabetics	Mean (sd) diabetics	T-test p-value	%mean difference	Cohen's d Effect
PSV baseline	56.3 (5.3)cm/s	73.0 (11.0)cm/s	<0.0001	16.2%	1.95
PSV 90 minutes	48.0 (5.1)cm/s	57.0 (8.1)cm/s	<0.0001	9.0%	1.30
PSV 150 minutes	47.0 (5.0)cm/s	54.1 (8.0)cm/s	<0.0001	7.2%	1.10
PSV 210minutes	44.0 (4)cm/s	45.2 (9)cm/s	0.4	1.2%	0.18

6.6.4 Peak systolic velocity change within groups at specific time points

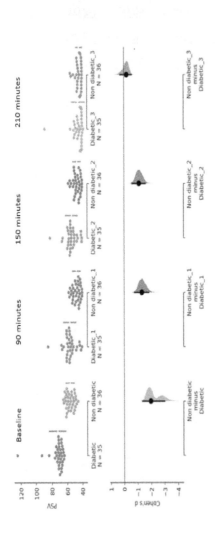

Figure 12 Shows peak systolic velocity change after beetroot ingestions within and between groups.

Key: PSV- Peak Systolic velocity

Within groups, peak systolic velocity decreased significantly and meaningfully ($P ≤ 0.0001$; $d ≤ 1.95$) at 90 minutes and 210 minutes after beetroot juice ingestions within diabetic patients and non-diabetic patients similarly. However, no significant or meaningful decrease ($p > 0.05$; $d ≤ 1.10$) occurred at 150 minutes time point after beetroot juice intake within both groups (figure 12; table 13).

Table 13 Comparison of peak systolic velocity changes at specific time points within groups.

Parameter	baseline	90 minutes	% mean difference	T-test p-value	Cohen's d effect size
Diabetic patients					
PSV	73.0 (11.0) cm/s	57.0 (8.1) cm/s	16.1%	<0.0001	1.70
	90 minutes	150 minutes			
	57.0 (8.1) cm/s	54.1 (8.0) cm/s	3.0%	0.2	0.29
	150 minutes	210 minutes			
	54.1 (8.0) cm/s	46.0 (9.0) cm/s	9%	<0.0001	1.08
Non - diabetic participants					
PSV	baseline	90 minutes	% mean Difference	T-test p-value	Cohen's d effect size
	56.3 (5.3) cm/s	47.0 (5.1)	9%	<0.0001	1.66
	90 minutes	150 minutes			
	47.0 (5.1) cm/s	47.0 (5.0)	1.0%	0.5	0.15
	150 minutes	210 minutes			
	47.0 (5.0) cm/s	44.0 (4.0) cm/s	3%	0.01	0.67

6.6.5 Combined groups systolic Blood pressure changes to beetroot juice ingestion at specific time points.

Combined group effects for systolic blood pressure showed a significant change between the baseline and 90 minutes time point *(diff = 13.0 mmHg; P <0.0001)*, baseline and 150 minutes time point *(diff = 14.3 mmHg; P = 0.0001)*; baseline and 210 minutes time point *(diff = 22.0; P <0.0001)* and between the 150 minutes to 210 minutes time point *(diff = 8.0 mmHg; P = 0.01)* after beetroot juice ingestions. However, there was no significant change in systolic blood pressure at the 90 minutes and 150 minutes time point *(diff = 1.2 mmHg; P = 1.00)* (Table 14).

Table 14: Combined group effects for systolic blood pressure changes after beetroot juice ingestion at specific time points (Benferroni).

	Baseline	90 minutes	150 minutes
90 minutes	-13.0 mmHg (diff) $P = 0.000$		
150 minutes	-14.3 mmHg (diff) $P = 0.000$	-1.2 mmHg (diff) $P = 1.000$	
210 minutes	-22.1 mmHg (diff) $P = 0.000$	-9.1 mmHg (diff) $P = 0.001$	-8.0 mmHg (diff) $P = 0.009$
Diff = mean difference; p = value			

6.6.6 Comparison of systolic blood pressure changes between groups at specific time points.

Systolic Blood Pressure was significantly and meaningfully higher ($P = 0.005$; $d = 0.68$) in the diabetic patients (156.0 ± 20.3 mmHg) compared to non-diabetic patients (143.1 ± 16.0 mmHg) basally. At 90 minutes after beetroot juice intake there was no significant/meaningful difference ($P > 0.05$; $d = 0.34$) in SBP between diabetic patients (139.0 ± 16.0 mmHg) and non-diabetic patients (134.0 ± 13.0 mmHg). At 150 minutes after beetroot juice intake, there was no significant or meaningful difference in SBP ($P > 0.05$; $d = 0.06$) between diabetic patients (135.4 ± 14.4 mmHg) and non-diabetic patients (135.0 ± 13.4 mmHg). At 210 minutes after beetroot juice intake again there was no significant or meaningful difference ($P > 0.05$; $d = 0.13$) between diabetic patients (128.0 ± 9.0 mmHg) and non-diabetic patients (127.0 ± 9.0 mmHg) (Table 15; Figure 13).

Table 15 Comparison of systolic blood pressure changes between groups at specific time points.

Parameter	Non - diabetics	Diabetics	T-test p value	% mean difference	Cohen's d effect sizes.
SBP baseline	143.1 (16.0) mmHg	156.0 (20.3) mmHg	0.01	12%	0.68
SBP 90 minutes	134.0 (13.0) mmHg	139.0 (16.0) mmHg	0.2	5.0%	0.34
SBP 150 minutes	135.0 (13.4) mmHg	135.4 (14.4) mmHg	1.0	1%	0.06
SBP 210 minutes	127.0 (9.0) mmHg	128.0 (9.0) mmHg	1.0	1.2%	0.13

6.6.7 Systolic Blood Pressure change within groups at specific time points.

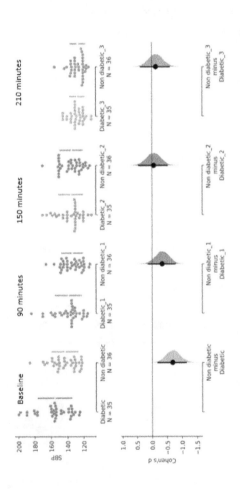

Figure 13 shows systolic blood pressure change after beetroot juice ingestions both within and between groups.

Key: SBP- Systolic Blood pressure

Within groups, systolic blood pressure reduced significantly and meaningfully ($P \leq 0.01$; $d \leq 0.92$) at 90 minutes and similarly at 210 minutes time point after beetroot juice ingestions within both the diabetic and the non-diabetic groups. However, no significant or meaningful decrease ($P > 0.05$; $d \leq 0.15$) occurred at 150 minutes after beetroot juice ingestions within both groups (figures 13; Table 16).

Table 16 Systolic Blood Pressure change within groups at specific time points.

	Diabetic participants				
SBP	baseline	90 minutes	%mean difference	T-test p-value	Cohen's d effect sizes
	156.0 (20.3) mmHg	139.0 (16.0) mmHg	17%	<0.001	0.92
	90 minutes	150 minutes			
	139.0 (16.0) mmHg	135.4 (14.4) mmHg	3.3%	0.4	0.22
	150 minutes	210 minutes			
	135.4 (14.4) mmHg	128.0 (9.0) mmHg	8.0%	0.01	0.64
	Non-diabetic participants				
SBP	baseline	90 minutes	%Mean difference	T-test p-value	Cohen's d effect sizes
	143.1(16.0) mmHg	134.0 (13.0) mmHg	9.3%	0.01	0.65
	90 minutes	150 minutes			
	134.0 (13.0) mmHg	135.0 (13.4) mmHg	0.8%	0.8	0.06
	150 minutes	210 minutes			
	135 (13.4) mmHg	127.0 (9.0) mmHg	8%	<0.0001	0.70

6.6.8 Combined groups diastolic blood pressure changes after beetroot juice ingestion at specific time points.

Combined group effects for diastolic blood pressure showed a significant change between the baseline and 90 minutes time point (diff = -7.1 mmHg; $P \leq 0.0001$), baseline and 150 minutes time point (diff = 8.4 mmHg; $P = 0.0001$); baseline and 210 minutes time point (diff = 13.4 mmHg; $P = 0.0001$) and between the 150 minutes and 210 minutes time point (diff = 5.0 mmHg; $P = 0.001$). However, there was no significant change in diastolic blood pressure between the 90 minutes and 150 minutes time point (diff = 1.3 mmHg; $P = 1.00$) after beetroot juice ingestions (Table 17).

Table 17 Combined groups' diastolic blood pressure changes after beetroot juice ingestion at specific time points (Benferroni).

	baseline	90 minutes	150 minutes
90 minutes	-7.1 mmHg (diff) P = 0.000		
150 minutes	-8.4 mmHg (diff) P = 0.000	-1.3 mmHg (diff) P = 1.000	
210 minutes	-13.4 mmHg P = 0.000	-6.3 mmHg (diff) P = 0.000	-5.0 mmHg (diff) P = 0.001
Diff = mean difference; p = value			

6.6.9 Comparison of diastolic blood pressure change at specific time points within groups.

Between groups, basal diastolic blood pressure did not show a significant/meaningful difference *(P>0.05; d = 0.33)* between diabetic patients *(101.0 ± 10.2 mmHg)* and non-diabetic patients *(98.0 ± 8.0 mmHg)*. At 90 minutes after beetroot juice intake there was no significant or meaningful difference (P >0.05; d = 0.08) between diabetic patients (92.0 ± 8.2 mmHg) and non-diabetic patients *(92.4 ± 7.2 mmHg)*. At 150 minutes after beetroot juice intake there was no significant or meaningful difference *(P >0.05; d = 0.08)* between diabetic patients *(91.0 ± 8.0 mmHg)* and non-diabetic patients (91.1 ± 7.0 mmHg). At 210 minutes after beetroot juice intake there was no significant or meaningful difference *(P >0.05; d = 0.23)* between diabetic patients *(86.4 ± 6.0 mmHg)* and non-diabetic patients *(85.2 ± 4.4 mmHg)* (Table 18; Figure 14).

Table 18 Comparison of diastolic blood pressure change between groups at specific time points.

Parameter	Non - diabetics	Diabetics	T-test p-value	% Mean difference	Cohen's d effect sizes
DBP baseline	98.0 (8.0) mmHg	100.7 (10.2) mmHg	0.2	3.1%	0.33
DBP 90mins	92.4 (7.2) mmHg	92.0 (8.2) mmHg	0.7	1.0%	0.08
DBP 150mins	91.1 (7.0) mmHg	90.5 (8.0) mmHg	0.7	0.6%	0.08
DBP 210mins	85.2 (4.4) mmHg	86.4 (6.0) mmHg	0.3	1.1%	0.23

6.6.10 Diastolic blood pressure changes within groups at specific time points.

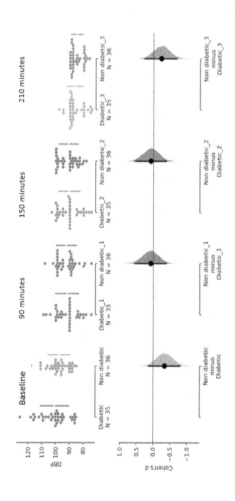

Figure 14 show diastolic blood pressure change within and between groups

Key: *DBP – Diastolic Blood Pressure*

Within groups, diastolic blood pressure decreased significantly and meaningfully (P ≤0.02; d ≤ 1.02) at 90 minutes and 210 minutes *after* beetroot juice ingestions within both groups. However, no significant/meaningful decrease (P >0.05; d ≤ 0.19) was seen at 90 minutes to 150 minutes after Beetroot juice ingestion by both groups (figure 14; table 19).

Table 19: shows a comparison of diastolic blood pressure changes at specific time points within groups.

	Non – diabetic participants				
DBP	baseline	90 minutes	% mean difference	T-test p-value	Cohen's d effect sizes
	98.0 (8.0) mmHg	92.4 (7.2) mmHg	5.3%	<0.0001	0.70
	90 minutes	150 minutes			
	92.1 (7.2) mmHg	91.1 (8.0) mmHg	1.4%	0.4	0.19
	150 minutes	210 minutes			
	91.0(8.0) mmHg	85.2 (4.4)mmHg	6.0%	<0.0001	1.02
	Diabetic participants				
DBP	baseline	90 minutes	% mean difference	T-test p-value	Cohen's d effect sizes
	101.0(10.3) mmHg	92.0(8.3) mmHg	9.0%	<0.0001	0.96
	90 minutes	150 minutes			
	92.0 (8.3) mmHg	90.5 (8.0)mmHg	1.3%	0.5	0.16
	150 minutes	210 minutes			
	90.5 (8.0)mmHg	86.4 mmHg	4.1%	0.02	0.60

6.7 Discussion

In this investigation, within groups, peak systolic velocity, systolic blood pressure and diastolic blood pressure reduced significantly and meaningfully from baseline to 90 minutes and from 150 minutes 210 minutes ($P \leq 0.01$; $d \leq 1.70$) after beetroot juice ingestion. However, no significant or meaningful change ($P > 0.05$; $d \leq 0.29$) occurred in peak systolic velocity, systolic blood pressure and diastolic blood pressure from 90 minutes to 150 minutes after beetroot juice ingestion.

The findings in this investigation suggested that short term effects of beetroot juice ingestion resulted in improved blood flow as reflected by reduced peak systolic velocity, systolic blood pressure and diastolic blood pressure in both groups across all time points after beetroot juice ingestion. Prior studies have been undertaken on assessing the short term effects of beetroot juice within an intervention period ranging from 3 hours to about 15 days and the acute effects established were on blood pressure and exercise endurance, while no prior studies were yet done on the effects of beetroot juice on blood flow using peak systolic velocity during the writing up of this book.

A study by Bahra et al., (2012), showed similar findings of improved vascular compliance signalling improved blood flow when conducted in hypertensive patients after ingestion of nitrate salts. Improved vascular compliance was reflected by a reduction in aortic pulse wave velocity and reduction in systolic blood pressure, while this investigation showed improved blood flow through reduced peak systolic velocity and reduction of blood pressure in diabetic patients and non-diabetic controls after ingestion of beetroot juice. These concurring findings justify the presence of a similar ingredient in beetroot juice and potassium nitrate salts which resulted in desirable improved blood flow effects in both hypertensive and diabetic patients.

The findings in this investigation showed improved blood flow in the asymptomatic diabetic patients and non-diabetic controls after 3 hours post beetroot juice ingestion as a clinically significant benefit and these findings prompted for long term assessment of chronic beetroot juice intake by diabetic patients with early-stage PAD as a post-doctoral study. Such improvements in blood flow if the long term could result in the reduction of medications needed to relieve impaired blood flow and those needed to reduce elevated blood pressure in diabetic patients. This improved blood flow after ingestion of beetroot juice carries the benefit of adaptation to exercise (Vanhatalo et al., 2010; Webb et al., 2008) and physical activity by patients with early-stage PAD thus improving their health management.

Between groups, peak systolic velocity and systolic blood pressure were significantly and meaningfully higher ($P \leq 0.04$; $d \leq 1.95$) in diabetic patients at baseline. However, at 90 minutes and 150 minutes peak systolic velocity remained higher in diabetic patients ($P \leq 0.04$; $d \leq 1.30$) unlike systolic blood pressure ($P > 0.05$; $d \leq 0.34$). At 210 minutes after beetroot juice ingestions peak systolic velocity and systolic blood pressure showed no significant or meaningful change in diabetics and non-diabetics ($P > 0.05$; $d \leq 0.18$). Diastolic blood pressure showed no significant or meaningful difference ($P > 0.05$; $d \leq 0.33$) between the groups at all the time points after beetroot juice ingestions.

Peak systolic velocity and systolic blood pressure showed a clinically significant change in blood between groups across all time points after intake of beetroot juice since their percentage (%) mean difference (less or equal to 22.1%) was higher than the smallest detectable difference (SDD %) from the first investigation (9.2%). However, diastolic blood pressure did not show a clinically significant change in blood flow between groups across all the time points since its percentage (%) mean difference (less or equal to 3.1%)) was lower than the smallest detectable difference (SDD %) from the first investigation (9.2%).

In the comparison for combined effects, peak systolic velocity showed a significant change (diff ≤ 19.7 cm/s; P ≤0.0001) between the baseline and 90 minutes, baseline and 150 minutes, baseline and 210 minutes, and finally 150 minutes and 210 minutes time points. However, there was no significant change in peak systolic velocity (diff = 0.4 cm/s; P = 1.00) between the 90 minutes and 150 minutes time point after beetroot juice ingestions. The combined effects for systolic blood pressure showed a significant change (diff ≤ 22.0 mmHg; P <0.0001) between baseline and 90 minutes, baseline and 150 minutes, baseline and 210 minutes and finally 150 minutes to 210 minutes time points after beetroot juice ingestions. However, there was no significant change in systolic blood pressure during the 90 minutes to 150 minutes time point (diff = 1.2 mmHg; P = 1.00). Diastolic blood pressure showed a significant change (diff ≤13.4 mmHg; P <0.0001) between baseline and 90 minutes, baseline and 150 minutes, baseline and 210 minutes, and 150 minutes and 210 minutes time points after beetroot juice ingestions. However, there was no significant change in diastolic blood pressure between the 90 minutes and 150 minutes time point (diff = 1.3 mmHg; P = 1.00) after beetroot juice ingestions.

These findings are in line with the research question of this study which sought to determine if the peak systolic velocity alongside systolic blood pressure and diastolic blood pressure were capable of demonstrating the acute effects of beetroot juice on blood flow within groups and between groups across time points while a significant and meaningful difference in blood flow was interpreted as the capability to show the acute effects of beetroot juice across the time points. The statistically significant and meaningful difference reflected by peak systolic, systolic blood pressure and diastolic blood pressure at 90 minutes after beetroot juice intake could be due to an increment in volume of blood after ingestion of 500 ml of beetroot juice while at 150 minutes after beetroot juice ingestions there was no significant change in peak systolic velocity, systolic blood pressure and diastolic blood pressure probably due to the continual flow of blood which brought back its volume to the baseline level. However, the significant and meaningful differences/ changes later noted in peak systolic velocity, systolic blood pressure and diastolic blood pressure during the 150 minutes – 210 minutes time point after beetroot juice ingestion could have been being the ones showing the true acute effects of the beetroot juice on the blood flow of the popliteal arteries of diabetic patients with early-stage PAD and non-diabetic controls.

Prior studies (Web et al., 2008; Bailey et al., 2009, 2010; Vanhatalo et al., 2010; Gilchrist et al., 2011; Lansely et al., 2011) have shown the effects of beetroot juice intake as reduced systolic blood pressure at least 3 hours post-ingestion and most of the studies were done in healthy normotensive individuals. During the writing up of this book, there was no prior study which showed the acute effects of beetroot juice ingestion on blood flow by utilising duplex ultrasound peak systolic velocity in individuals who were at greater cardiovascular risk (Siervo et al., 2013; Ogbonmwan et al., 2012). This investigation has shown the evidence of improved blood flow as reflected by reduced peak systolic velocity and reduced systolic blood pressure and diastolic blood pressure during the 2 ½ -3 ½ hours' time point in individuals at a greater risk of cardiovascular disease (diabetic patients with early-stage PAD) after ingestion of beetroot juice.

Beetroot juice studies have confirmed the bioavailability of nitrite and nitric oxide from the nitrate in beetroot juice as being at less or equal to 3 hrs (180 minutes) -post-ingestion (Kapil et al., 2010; Kenjale et al., 2011; Webb et al., 2008; Vanhatalo et al., 2010). Similarly in this investigation, peak systolic velocity, diastolic blood pressure and systolic blood pressure showed a significant difference in blood flow both in diabetic patients and non-diabetic patients from 150 minutes to 210 minutes (2 ½ - 3 ½ hours) time point after beetroot juice ingestion.

In this investigation, the fact that no significant or meaningful difference was found between groups after 210 minutes (3 ½ hours) could also mean the peak presence of the acute effects of beetroot juice in the blood for both groups. These findings could be owed to the peak bioavailability of nitrite and nitric oxide in the bloodstream after digestion and excretion of the beetroot juice nitrate (Kapil et al., 2010, Kenjale et al., 2011).

This investigation noted a reduction in the peak systolic velocity of the popliteal arteries in diabetic patients *(73.0 ± 11.0 cm/s pre to 45.2 ± 9.0 cm/s during 2 ½ to 3 ½ hrs post 500ml beetroot juice ingestion; p< 0.05)* and a reduction of peak systolic velocity in the popliteal arteries of non-diabetic patients *(57.0 ± 5.3 cm/s pre to 44 ± 4.0 cm/s during 2 ½ to 3 ½ hours post beetroot juice ingestion)*. Similarly, this investigation also noted a reduction in systolic blood pressure in diabetic patients with early-stage PAD *(156.0 ± 20.3 mmHg pre to 128.0 ± 9.0 mmHg during 2 ½ -3 ½ hours post-Beetroot Juice intake; p < 0.05)* and a reduction in non-diabetic controls *(143.4 ± 16.0 mmHg pre to 127.0 ± 9.0 mmHg during 2 ½ -3 ½ hours post-Beetroot Juice ingestion, p < 0.05)*. Concurring with these findings, other studies (Hobbs et al., 2012; Kapil et al., 2015) also noted a reduction in systolic blood pressure *(% mean difference = 20.5%)* and a reduction in diastolic blood pressure *(% mean difference = 14.6%)* at about 2 - 3 hours post-ingestion of 5.7 mmol beetroot juice. However a reduction in pulse wave velocity in hypertensive patients after dietary nitrate consumption by 0.59 m/s *(95% CI 0.2 - 0.9; p < 0.01)* compared to baseline values and 0.6 m/s *(95% CI 0.1 - 1.1; p <0.05)* compared to placebo was shown by Kapil et al., 2015).

6.8 Strengths and limitations.

The strength of this investigation was that the principal investigator carried it out under controlled settings and which limited transfer, recall, selection and misclassification of exposure factors bias and measurement error. An example was the objective selection of diabetic patients with early-stage PAD using reactive hyperaemic testing and also the prior preparations by participants before the undertaking of blood pressure and blood flow measurements and the beetroot juice intervention. Prior studies assessing the effects of beetroot juice (Kenjale et al., 2011; Kapil et al., 2010; Vanhatalo et al., 2011; Webb et al., 2008; Bailey et al., 2010) accordingly put such similar measures and controls in place.

Performance bias was limited during the gathering of data since the same principal investigator holding more than 5 years' experience in vascular ultrasound imaging is the one who performed the duplex ultrasound and blood pressure measurements in this investigation while blinded to the final collation of these findings with the participants' anonymously coded demographic data which was undertaken by the research assistants.

Recall bias was limited since principal investigator measured values for ultrasound parameters and blood pressure and stored them in the archives of the sonar machine but was blinded to the collation of these values with the participants' anonymous codes and this was done by the research assistants. The control measures (Kapil et al., 2010; Vanhatalo et al., 2011) utilised in this book also contributed to effective screening for the sample of asymptomatic diabetic patients with early-stage PAD for this investigation and thus minimising bias due to misclassification of exposure and outcomes, while prior patient preparations also allowed basal blood flow to be similar in all participants before the ingestion of the beetroot juice intervention to reduce measurement error.

The principal investigator made the following decisions which resulted as weaknesses in the third and final investigation of this book;

i) Dropping further assessment of the dorsalis pedis artery during the first investigation due to lack of reproducibility of the vessel diameter inner to inner measurements.

ii) Dropping pulsatility index from further analysis in the third investigation due to reasons of increased variability displayed in the second investigation.

iii) Dropping, resistive index from further assessment in the third investigation despite it coming out as robust in the second investigation to enable a more focussed assessment of peak systolic velocity in assessing acute effects of beetroot juice in the popliteal arteries only since the blood flow effects quickly waned away in this investigation.

The three decisions made by the principal investigator after the first and second investigations then resulted in this investigation showing findings of the acute effects of beetroot juice in the popliteal arteries only with the exclusion of the posterior tibial and anterior tibial arteries while peak systolic velocity was the only duplex ultrasound parameter which was finally utilised in this investigation alongside systolic blood pressure and diastolic blood pressure. Therefore, the principal investigator will determine findings for the resistive index in the anterior tibial and posterior tibial arteries later in post-doctoral studies.

6.9 Internal and external validity

The budget for this investigation was limited such that the principal investigator could not afford to draw a wider heterogeneous sample which could include other populations resident in Zimbabwe to justify its external validity and generalisability to the whole Zimbabwean population. However, the principal investigator put in place a tight inclusion and exclusion criteria thus the investigation had high internal validity and the findings could be generalised to the Zimbabwean Black/African population of asymptomatic diabetic patients with early-stage PAD and the non-diabetic controls. However, external validity was limited in this investigation since the sample was not heterogeneous and did not include other populations resident in Zimbabwe besides Black/Africans.

6.10 Conclusions

The findings of this investigation concluded that the acute effects of beetroot juice in the popliteal arteries of Black/African asymptomatic diabetic patients with early-stage PAD and non-diabetic controls reflected as reduced peak systolic velocity, systolic blood pressure and diastolic blood pressure during the 150 - 210 minutes time point. However, peak systolic velocity also showed a clinically significant change in blood flow between groups which was not shown by systolic blood pressure and diastolic blood pressure.

6.11 Recommendations

From the findings of this investigation, the principal investigator recommended the ingestion of beetroot juice by asymptomatic diabetic patients with early-stage PAD and non-diabetic participants to enable improved blood flow and better management of blood pressure. However, the principal investigator will need to augment these findings after the undertaking of post-doctoral work assessing the long term effects of beetroot juice ingestion by these diabetic patients who are at a greater risk for cardiovascular diseases.

The principal investigator also recommended the utilisation of duplex ultrasound peak systolic velocity to monitor long term effects of beetroot juice ingestion by asymptomatic diabetic patients after it demonstrated a clinically significant and meaningful change in blood flow between groups in this investigation.

6.12 Implications

The findings of this investigation imply that the acute effects of beetroot juice ingestion result in improved blood flow and reduced blood pressure as reflected by duplex ultrasound peak systolic velocity, systolic blood pressure and diastolic blood pressure.

The findings of this investigation showed that ingestion of beetroot juice resulted in clinically significant changes in blood flow as demonstrated by peak systolic velocity thereby implying that beetroot juice ingestion has short term therapeutic effects in both diabetic patients as well as non-diabetic controls which may need pursuing in long term ingestion of beetroot juice.

6.13 Decision making for areas of future research (post-doctoral)

The principal investigator decided to undertake a longitudinal multi-centre post-doctoral study which embraces a heterogeneous Zimbabwean population. This study will pursue the long term effects of beetroot juice ingestion by asymptomatic diabetic patients with early-stage PAD and non-diabetic controls using duplex ultrasound peak systolic velocity and resistive index together with blood pressure measurements to improve on the external validity and generalisability of these findings to the Zimbabwean population.

Chapter 7 - Overall book discussion

7.1 Introduction

The principal investigator carried out the methodology of this book as three separate experimental investigations which built into each other. In the first investigation, the principal investigator determined the repeatability of the duplex ultrasound parameters in measuring lower limb blood flow in 10 asymptomatic diabetic patients with early-stage PAD. In this first investigation repeatability of duplex ultrasound parameters was quantified through the determination of their within and between sessions reliability and measurement error. The findings of the first investigation established duplex ultrasound peak systolic velocity, pulsatility index and resistive index as robust parameters with the exclusion of vessel diameter inner to inner in the measurement of blood flow in the popliteal arteries, posterior tibial arteries and anterior tibial arteries.

In the second investigation, the principal investigator determined the robustness of the statistically significant ultrasound parameters from the first investigation in demonstrating the effects of early-stage PAD on the lower limb blood flow of 35 diabetic patients and non-diabetic controls. The findings of the second investigation established peak systolic velocity and resistive index as the robust duplex ultrasound parameters in demonstrating the effects of early-stage PAD in the popliteal arteries, anterior tibial arteries and posterior tibial arteries except for pulsatility index.

In the third investigation, the principal investigator determined the effects of beetroot juice ingestion on the lower limb arteries blood flow of the two groups of participants imported from the second investigation using the emerging robust peak systolic velocity from the second investigation together with systolic and diastolic blood pressure across three-time points thus the baseline – 90 minutes; 90 minutes – 150 minutes; and finally the 150 minutes – 210 minutes. The findings of the third investigation established the acute effects of beetroot juice ingestion as reduced blood pressure and improved blood flow in the popliteal arteries of asymptomatic diabetic patients with early-stage PAD and non-diabetic controls.

7.2 Overall book Findings

The first investigation of this book showed that the ultrasound parameters consisting of peak systolic velocity, pulsatility index and resistive index were repeatable in assessing blood flow in the lower limb arteries of diabetics with early-stage PAD due to their demonstration of good to excellent reliability, low variability and an acceptably low standard error of measurement (SEM) and smallest detectable difference (SDD %) except for vessel diameter inner to inner. The findings of the first investigation of this book concurred with the findings of prior reliability studies which have shown minimum variability low SEM (Thomas et al., 2015; Sheppard et al., 2011) as well as good to excellent reliability (Koo and Lee, 2016). Eiberg et al., (2010) showed an acceptable magnitude of the measurement error and reliability of duplex ultrasound in diabetic patients with late-stage PAD. However, no evidence was found on the assessment of the repeatability of duplex ultrasound parameters in measuring blood flow in diabetic patients with early-stage PAD during the writing of this book. Thus, the findings of this book have indicated justifiable evidence on the robustness of duplex ultrasound parameters in measuring effects of early-stage PAD on blood flow in Black/African Zimbabwean asymptomatic diabetic patients. Duplex ultrasound is the cheapest imaging modality which is readily available in secondary care settings of district hospitals in Zimbabwe, thus the greater population of diabetic patients may be afforded earlier assessments for PAD more cheaply and affordably.

Findings for the second investigation of this book showed that amongst the robust duplex ultrasound parameters from the first investigation, peak systolic velocity and resistive index were capable of demonstrating the effects of early-stage PAD on the lower limb arterial blood flow of diabetic patients with the exclusion of pulsatility index. The findings of the second investigation provided justifiable evidence to utilise duplex ultrasound peak systolic velocity and resistive index when screening for early-stage PAD to augment the findings of the already recommended Ankle Brachial Index.

Findings for the third investigation of this book showed justifiable evidence on the robustness of duplex ultrasound peak systolic velocity alongside systolic blood pressure and diastolic blood pressure in demonstrating the acute effects of beetroot juice ingestion on the blood flow of the popliteal arteries of diabetic patients with early-stage PAD and non-diabetic controls. The findings of the third investigation showed the clinically significant acute effects of beetroot juice ingestion as reduced blood pressure and improved blood flow in the popliteal arteries of these participants during the 2 ½ -3 ½ hours' time point as demonstrated by peak systolic velocity. In the third investigation of this book, the acute effects of beetroot juice were demonstrated during the 2 ½ -3 ½ hours' time slot which coincided with the same time (less or equal to 3 hours) for the bioavailability of nitrite and nitric oxide from the nitrate of ingested beetroot juice which reflected as reduced blood pressure (Kenjale et al., 2011; Webb et al., 2008; Vanhatalo et al., 2010; Kapil et al.,2010), enhanced exercise performance (Vanhatalo et al., 2010; Webb et al., 2008; Kenjale et al., 2011), peaking plasma nitrite (Kenjale et al., 2011).

The Ankle Brachial Index test was performed in all the participants for the first and second investigations as a parallel test since prior evidence has shown Ankle Brachial Index being popularly recommended to screen and quantify asymptomatic PAD (Hirsh et al., 2005; Norgren et al. 2007; Gerhard-Herman et al., 2006; Rooke et al., 2011) while there were no prior studies done to show justifying evidence to recommend the utilisation of duplex ultrasound in assessing early-stage PAD in asymptomatic participants during the writing up of this book. Prior evidence in other populations has shown normal range levels of Ankle Brachial Index of greater or equal to 0.9 and less or equal to 1 while values less than 0.9 would indicate the presence of PAD and values greater than 1.3 would indicate incompressible arteries with median calcification in diabetic patients, (Chen et al, 2015; Park et al, 2012; Jude, 2004). In this book, the mean Ankle Brachial Index for the participants in both groups was normal range 1.1 (± 0.1) justifying that the diabetic patients in this book did not have symptomatic/late-stage PAD but early-stage /asymptomatic PAD instead.

7.3 Overall contribution to knowledge gap.

Firstly, this book has contributed to the existing gap in knowledge that the duplex ultrasound parameters such peak systolic velocity, pulsatility index and resistive index are robust measures with low measurement error in the assessment of lower limb arterial blood flow in asymptomatic diabetic patients with early-stage PAD (first investigation).

Secondly, this book contributed new knowledge that clinically significant effects of early-stage PAD on lower limb arterial blood flow of diabetic patients can be demonstrated by duplex ultrasound peak systolic velocity and resistive index (second investigation).

Thirdly this book contributed new knowledge that the acute effects of beetroot juice ingestion on lower limb arterial blood flow of diabetic patients with early-stage PAD and non-diabetic controls were demonstrated as reduced peak systolic velocity and reduced systolic and diastolic blood pressure during the 2 ½ -3 ½ hours' time point post beetroot juice ingestion. Again, Peak systolic velocity demonstrated a clinically significant change in blood flow between groups 2 ½ -3 ½ hours post beetroot juice ingestion which could be interpreted as therapeutic (third investigation).

7.4 Overall book conclusions

Based on the findings of the three studies of this book, the principal investigator made the following conclusions;

i) The first investigation

The duplex ultrasound peak systolic velocity, pulsatility index and resistive index are a robust measuring tool for lower limb arterial blood flow in Zimbabwean Black/African diabetic patients with early-stage (asymptomatic) PAD except for vessel diameter inner to inner.

ii) The second investigation

The duplex ultrasound peak systolic velocity and resistive index are capable of demonstrating the effects of early-stage PAD on the lower limb arteries blood flow of Zimbabwean Black/African asymptomatic diabetic patients with the exclusion of pulsatility index.

iii) The third investigation

The duplex ultrasound peak systolic velocity alongside systolic blood pressure and diastolic blood pressure demonstrated the acute effects of beetroot juice ingestion as improved blood flow and reduced blood pressure respectively during the 2 ½ and 3 ½ hours post beetroot juice ingestion in Zimbabwean Black/African diabetic patients and non-diabetic controls. Peak systolic velocity demonstrated clinical significant blood flow change between groups post beetroot juice ingestion, which is likely due to vasodilation.

7.5 Overall implications of book findings

From the findings of this book the principal investigator deducted the following implications;

i) Duplex ultrasound peak systolic velocity and resistive index are robust parameters to measure and quantify the effects of early-stage PAD on the lower limb arterial blood flow of Zimbabwean Black/African asymptomatic diabetic patients.

ii) The acute effects of beetroot juice ingestion by Zimbabwean Black/African diabetes can be demonstrated by duplex ultrasound peak systolic velocity alongside systolic and diastolic blood pressure. Peak systolic velocity can demonstrate short term therapeutic effects of beetroot juice ingestion by Zimbabwean Black/African asymptomatic diabetic patients and non-diabetic controls.

iii) This book findings have provided evidence which could be utilised to enhance earlier detection of the effects of early-stage PAD on the lower limb arterial blood flow of asymptomatic diabetic patients more cheaply and affordably in Zimbabwe.

iv) The background on the management of diabetes mellitus in Zimbabwe has indicated that the main drawbacks to effectively manage it was the shortage of basic commodities which include essential medicines and glucostrips (Parirenyatwa and Gwinji, 2016-2020). The results presented in this book provide evidence of improved blood flow and reduced blood pressure at 2 ½ -3 ½ hours post beetroot juice ingestion by diabetic patients and the non-diabetic controls and the fact that the demonstrated blood flow change effects were clinically significant could mean beetroot juice could be offering some form of therapy to these patients. It is suggested that Zimbabwean diabetic patients or non-diabetic controls should include more nitrate-rich vegetables, such as beetroot, in their diets to improve blood flow and reduce blood pressure. The benefit of reduced blood pressure and improvement in blood flow evidenced in the third investigation of this book are more favourable for 'normal' exercise-induced responses, which may further benefit the health of this population. However, additional post-doctoral research will be conducted to determine the chronic effects of beetroot juice ingestion and to determine if there will be additive benefits to increased physical activity.

v) A modified diet of nitrate-rich vegetables and a lifestyle of exercise can provide the Zimbabwean diabetic population with the benefit of reducing the burden of non-affordability of essential medications for improved blood flow and high blood pressure. Prior studies have also indicated that a sustaining control of blood pressure is only achieved in about 50% of hypertensive cases (Culter et al., 2008; Egan et al., 2010). This means that dietary based interventions are recognised as important strategies for primary prevention of high blood pressure (Savica et al., 2010) to reduce cardiovascular disease risk for example in diabetic patients.

7.6 Overall book recommendations

From the findings of this book, the principal investigator made the following recommendations;

i) A more liberal duplex assessment of the lower limb blood flow in asymptomatic diabetic patients should be enhanced in Zimbabwean secondary healthcare settings to enable early diagnosis of PAD.

ii) The findings of this book recommend a longitudinal study post-doctoral to determine the long term effects of beetroot juice ingestion on blood flow and blood pressure on multi-centre heterogeneous samples in Zimbabwe increase external validity for justifying these therapeutic effects to the Zimbabwean population.

7.7 Dissemination of book findings

The principal investigator will publish the results of this book in aggregate form, from which individuals will not be identifiable and there will be no personally identifying data. The principal investigator will present the first publication of this book as a PhD book in the University of Salford Doctoral school repository. Currently, this PhD book has three papers in the pipeline and the principal investigator plans to publish them as follows;

i) First investigation findings contributed to the existing literature review gap about the robustness of ultrasound parameters in measuring blood flow in the lower limbs of diabetic patients with early-stage PAD (Eiberg et al., 2010; Rooke et al., 2011). Therefore, the findings of this first investigation justify the repeatability of ultrasound parameters including peak systolic velocity, pulsatility index and resistive index in the measurement of blood flow in the lower limbs of asymptomatic diabetic patients with early-stage PAD. The findings from this first investigation may sensitise practising Zimbabwean sonographers and radiographers to utilise duplex ultrasound parameters when assessing blood flow in the diabetic patients, thus they will be published in the Zimbabwe Journal of Sciences Technology (ZJST). ZJST is open access, online and peer-reviewed journal published by the National University of Science and Technology, Zimbabwe with a coverage of about 74% in Zimbabwe and Africa (https://www.nust.ac.zw/ZJST/).

ii) The second investigation findings contributed to the existing literature review gap in the current practising guidelines (Rooke et al., 2011; Gerhard-Herman et al., 2016; Hirsh et al., 2005) where Ankle Brachial Index has been solely recommended for the quantification and screening of early-stage PAD in asymptomatic diabetic patients. The findings of the second investigation of this book justify the ability of duplex ultrasound peak systolic velocity and resistive index in quantifying the effects of early-stage PAD on the lower limb blood flow of Zimbabwean Black/African asymptomatic diabetic patients. Therefore the principal investigator plans to publish these findings in the Radiography journal. The Radiography journal is an open-access peer-reviewed medical journal published by Elsevier which covers diagnostic and therapeutic radiography and having a high impact factor of 0.74 (https://www.journals.elsevier.com/radiography). The radiography journal commands a wide readership in the Radiography community, in Europe, Africa and beyond. Therefore, the principal investigator chose this journal as a suitable channel to promote the dissemination of this knowledge to sonographers and radiographers practising ultrasound to augment the findings of Ankle Brachial Index with ultrasound parameters during the screening and quantification of PAD in asymptomatic diabetic patients.

iii) The findings of the third investigation of this book justified improvement of blood flow and reduction of blood pressure after about 2 ½ hrs post-ingestion of beetroot juice by asymptomatic diabetic patients. This evidence was measured by duplex ultrasound peak systolic velocity and blood pressure where clinically significant changes were detected and this suggested some therapeutic effects of beetroot juice ingestion. These findings were generalised to the population of the diabetic Zimbabwean Black/Africans of which most of them reside in poor communities and rural areas. In this case, the principal investigator will use the local ZJST to disseminate this evidence to the intellectual Zimbabwean and African community. However, to reach out to the ordinary rural population, the principal investigator plans to book a health and fitness talk show slot with Radio Zimbabwe, which is a radio station that broadcasts widely in the multi-languages spoken in Zimbabwe including the popular languages of Shona and Ndebele (www.radioZim.co.zw). To reach out to the wider urban and English speaking Zimbabwean community the principal investigator will book a health and fitness talk show with classic 263 radio station which broadcasts mainly in English to the mature audience of the urban population of Zimbabwe (https://www.classic 263.co.zw).

7.8 Appendices

Appendix A)

Data collection sheet for diabetics/non-diabetics participants for investigations 1 and 2

Participant code	e. g. DM01			
Age				
Gender				
ABI value				
Body mass index				
HbA$_{1c}$				
EGFR				
Reactive hyperaemic test	Normal ☐		abnormal ☐	
	Duplex ultrasound parameters			
Arterial level	PSV	PI	RI	VDI
PA				
ATA				
PTA				
DPA				

Appendix B

Data collection sheet for the third investigation.

Patient code			
Time Slots	SBP	DBP	PSV
Basal -1½ hours			
1½hrs - 2 ½ hours			
2 ½ hrs – 3 ½ hours			